Type 2 Turnaround

From Diagnosis to Dynamic Living

by
William Frye SR.

Table of Contents

Introduction:
Embracing the Journey Ahead

Life often presents us with unexpected challenges, moments that redefine our path and test the very fabric of our resilience. A diagnosis of type 2 diabetes can be one such pivotal moment, a juncture where the road ahead might seem daunting, shrouded in the unknown. Yet within each challenge lies an opportunity, a chance to embrace a journey that can lead to profound personal growth and well-being. This journey is not about a destination, but rather a transformation of lifestyle, perspective, and spirit.

Embarking on this path, you may find yourself facing a cascade of questions, concerns, and decisions. It's a natural reaction to the complex nature of diabetes, a condition that requires continuous learning and adaptation. But take heart—this journey is one you needn't walk alone. Let this book be a steadfast companion, illuminating the path ahead with information, strategies, and encouragement tailored to your needs.

The wisdom imparted by the ages tells us there is a season for everything under the heavens—a time to plant and a time to uproot, a time to tear down and a time to build. Your diagnosis could be seen as a time for both planting new habits and uprooting those that no longer serve you. It's a time to build a lifestyle that nurtures your body, mind, and spirit. In these times, we find new strength, and often, a new direction that leads us to a place of greater health and peace.

Just as a house built upon a rock stands firm, so too must your resolve as you manage your diabetes. Understanding what type 2 diabetes is, how it affects your body, and what risk factors contribute to it, will be the bedrock upon which your journey rests. This foundational knowledge equips you to make informed decisions and take control of your health.

Walking through the valley of diagnosis can stir a tempest of emotions. It's a time that tests the soul but remember that even in the darkest of times, there flickers a light of hope. With each step forward—each positive action you take—you will emerge stronger. Crafting your support team, those who will walk with you, is paramount. They are the friends who lift your arms when the battle tires you, your confidants who listen, and professionals who guide you with expertise.

Gone are the days of manna from heaven, but that doesn't mean your nutritional path needs to be barren. Creating a diabetes-friendly diet is akin to cultivating a garden that provides nourishment and vitality. Learning to decipher food labels and planning meals isn't just about food; it's about empowering yourself to make choices that support your health.

Remember, the body is a temple, and caring for it through exercise is both a stewardship and a celebration of life's capabilities. Exercise is more than movement; it's a potent medicine that strengthens the body and the will. It's not just about the type of exercise, but the joy and routine that come with it. Monitoring your progress, like a faithful gardener, ensures that your efforts are nurturing you in full.

Medications are tools, not crutches; they are designed to work with you, not for you. Mastering medication and glucose monitoring helps you maintain balance, akin to the skilled hand of a craftsman ensuring his work is true. Adjustments are part of the journey, a sign of responsiveness and care, not failure.

Our lives are not just reflected in the mirror, but also in the scales. Weight management isn't solely about aesthetics; it's a meaningful chapter in the story of your diabetes management. Strategies for tackling weight issues are not about quick fixes but sustainable practices that honor your body's needs.

In your daily sojourn, routine is your rhythm, the steady beat to which you can manage the highs and lows. Travel and sickness are part of life's journey, and having strategies to cope with such days imbues you with confidence and preparedness. It's your staff in hand as you traverse uncertain landscapes.

Yet this journey is not solely physical. Your mental health is like the still waters by which you must sometimes rest. Coping with burnout, managing emotions, and fostering resilience are essential to maintaining your inner peace and well-being. Your mental health is as crucial as your physical health; both require care and attention.

While you navigate this path, complications may sometimes look like Goliaths to your David. But equipped with knowledge, regular check-ups, and self-care practices like diligent foot and eye care, you become more than a match for these giants. Prevention is a shield carried in the foresight of taking each day as it comes.

Life is not lived in isolation, and diabetes will intersect with the lives of those you hold dear. A tapestry of relationships, from your family to friends, weaves around you, providing strength and color to your life. Educating them, sharing with them, and navigating the social aspects of life with diabetes enriches your experience and theirs.

Stewardship of resources is a Biblical principle that holds true for managing the costs associated with diabetes care. Understanding the financial terrain, from insurance to medication costs, can seem as daunting as facing an army with just a sling. Yet, strategies and assistance programs are like stones that can be fitly slung to hit their mark, enabling you to manage diabetes without financial ruin.

Finally, never lose hope for the future. Innovations in diabetes care keep the horizon bright with promises of new treatments and better management tools. Engaging with the latest technology and research is like drawing upon ancient wisdom—it offers insight, hope, and pathways to progress.

As you hold this book in your hands, consider it a map to the many facets of your journey. With each chapter, you'll gain insights not just into diabetes but into the measure of your courage and capacity for change. Embrace the journey ahead with an open heart and spirit, for through it you will not only manage diabetes—you will discover the fullness of life that comes from overcoming, learning, and thriving.

Chapter 1:
Understanding Type 2 Diabetes

In the wake of embracing our journey ahead, let us delve into the heart of the matter: Understanding Type 2 Diabetes. This is not merely an illness, but a call to a deeper understanding of our bodies and the delicate balance within. Type 2 diabetes unfolds when the body can't effectively use insulin, the herald that allows glucose to enter the cells and generate energy. This imbalance leads to elevated blood sugar levels, a silent tide that, over time, can erode the treasured shores of our health. Knowing the factors that contribute to this condition, such as genetics, lifestyle choices, and even the environment, is pivotal in navigating the waters ahead. It's also essential to recognize the early whispers of warning—those signs that may fleetingly appear and prompt us to action. Understanding these elements can empower us, providing a foundation upon which we can build healthier lives, fortified against the whims of this ailment. With informed minds and vigilant hearts, we can live in concert with diabetes, transforming what might be perceived as adversity into a testament of our resilience.

What Is Type 2 Diabetes? In our journey through understanding Type 2 diabetes, it is paramount to recognize the essence of what we face. Type 2 diabetes is a chronic condition that affects the way the body processes blood sugar, known as glucose. It is a battle not against the self, but with the self, akin to the trials that refine gold—making what is good into something even more precious.

At the heart of this condition is a resistance to insulin—a hormone critical for the regulation of blood glucose levels. Insulin is a key which unlocks cells, allowing them to absorb glucose and convert it into energy. In Type 2 diabetes, the cells begin to ignore the presence of insulin. This resistance prompts the pancreas to produce more insulin in an attempt to elicit a response, but over time, this gland tires and produces less insulin, resulting in elevated blood glucose levels.

While Type 1 diabetes is often linked with an inability to produce insulin due to an autoimmune response, Type 2 is largely influenced by lifestyle choices, genetics, and environmental factors. It is a silent reminder that our bodies are temples deserving of care and attention, echoing biblical wisdom that teaches us to steward our health with prudent diligence.

Many people walk with Type 2 diabetes for years without noticing, as symptoms can be as subtle as a whisper in a bustling market. It isn't a shout for attention, but a gradual shift where increased thirst, frequent urination, and unanticipated weight loss begin to paint a picture of an underlying condition that impacts every aspect of one's temple.

The prevalence of this condition in our modern society cannot be overstated. Millions are walking the same path, and while it can seem that the road is trodden in solitude, it's a shared journey. This commonality serves as a beacon of community and mutual support. Though the responsibility of daily management lies within the individual, the collective wisdom of those who walk before us lightens the load.

Blood sugar levels are more than numbers on a monitor; they tell a story of balance and harmony within our body. The aim is not just to maintain this harmony but to flourish in it, allowing ourselves to live abundantly, harkening back to the principle that life is to be lived in its fullness, with every day being a testament to perseverance and courage.

Type 2 diabetes is intimately linked with metabolic syndrome—a cluster of conditions including high blood pressure, high blood sugar, excess body fat around the waist, and abnormal cholesterol levels. These companions, though unwelcome, remind us that our health is interconnected, as a tapestry woven with various threads, each affecting the other.

Understanding this condition is to arm oneself with knowledge, wielded as a sword to cut through misconceptions. It's not a disease of character or a punishment for past choices but a medical challenge that can be met with grace and strength. It teaches that while we may not choose our trials, we can choose our response to them.

The management of Type 2 diabetes is as much about medical intervention as it is about lifestyle adaptation. Medications such as Metformin may enter one's story, but they are but one chapter in a much larger narrative—one filled with nourishment, physical movement, and mental well-being.

Being informed that one has Type 2 diabetes can be akin to arriving at a fork in the road. It presents an opportunity for transformation, inviting individuals to reevaluate their journey and take steps towards a destination of wellness. It's a call to adventure, one that asks for courage but promises growth.

To live with Type 2 diabetes is to learn to listen—to the signs of your body, to the advice of healthcare professionals, and to the testimonies of those who share in the same struggle. It requires the wisdom to know when to rest and when to push forward, reflecting understanding that our bodies are both temporal and resilient.

This condition asks of you to be a steward of your own health, to walk a path that is mindful of nutritional intake, conscious of physical activity, and sensitive to the whispers of your body that, when heeded, can prevent the shouts of complications down the road.

Indeed, Type 2 diabetes is not the end but a new beginning. It calls upon the human spirit to rise and adapt, to embrace the challenge as an opportunity to remake oneself. Like the phoenix rising from the ashes, a diagnosis can lead to a powerful reawakening of purpose and health.

Living with Type 2 diabetes isn't about lamenting over lost sweet treats—it's the joy of discovering a lifestyle that can be as rich and fulfilling as any other. With every healthy choice, every informed decision, you are rewriting your story, proving that with knowledge, wisdom, and determination, one's quality of life can soar even in the face of chronic illness.

In coming to grips with Type 2 diabetes, you embark on a deeply personal journey that can, in time, reveal inner strengths previously untapped. It's a refining process, where the hardships faced serve to strengthen character, deepen empathy, and cultivate a life lived in awareness and intentionality.

The Role of Insulin and Blood Sugar As we've delved into the nature of type 2 diabetes, it's clear that understanding the interplay of insulin and blood sugar is crucial. It's not simply a matter of knowing that insulin manages blood sugar levels; it's unraveling how this process affects your entire being. In the midst of life's stormy seas, acknowledging how insulin operates can be your beacon of hope, guiding you towards calmer waters and a more serene journey with diabetes.

In the beginning, God created all living things with remarkable precision and intricacy. The human body is no exception, designed to maintain balance or homeostasis. Insulin, a hormone produced by the pancreas, is part of this intricate design. It regulates the amount of glucose in the bloodstream, ensuring our cells receive the energy they need to thrive. Your body's ability to harness the energy from your meals is akin to the wisdom of Solomon—discerning and perfectly balanced.

However, in type 2 diabetes, this harmonious system encounters trials. The body's cells begin to resist insulin's message, much like a hardened heart resists wisdom's call. This resistance prompts the pancreas to produce more insulin in an attempt to restore order, yet over time, it can't keep up. Elevated blood sugar levels become the Goliath in this fight—a giant that seems insurmountable, but not undefeatable.

Understanding this condition requires not just knowledge but wisdom, for beyond the physical realm there is a spirit that must also be nourished. You are more than your diagnosis. You are a vessel of potential, capable of learning, adapting, and overcoming—to rise like a phoenix from the ashes of outdated habits and soar on the wings of renewed health and vitality.

Managing blood sugar isn't solely about medication or insulin therapy, though these can be essential components. It's about the integration of lifestyle changes—a daily breaking of bread wherein what you feed your body and soul becomes a testament to your resolve. The foods you choose, the exercises you engage in, these are like parables that, when lived, speak volumes about your dedication to life's beautiful tapestry.

Yet, even with discipline and understanding, blood sugar levels can sometimes be as unpredictable as the weather—changing with stress, illness, or even the unpredictable rhythm of life. Monitoring your glucose becomes as essential as the watchman in the night, ever vigilant, ensuring the city—your body—remains safe and secure.

Insulin therapy may become a part of your journey if lifestyle modifications and oral medications don't sufficiently manage blood sugar levels. If so, embrace it as you would a trusted friend who supports and aids you through trying times. Initial fears or disappointments can transform into strength and confidence, as David facing Goliath, with your sling being knowledge and your stone, unyielding resolve.

It is essential to see that this journey with blood sugar and insulin is not intended to be walked alone. Let healthcare providers be your council of elders, offering wisdom and guidance. Heed their advice as you would the wise words of prophets—champions of health guiding you to a promised land of well-being and balance.

Indeed, the road may be long, and at times you may falter like the Israelites in the wilderness, questioning if the promised land is within reach. Remember then, as now, that perseverance brings forth character, and character, hope—a hope that does not disappoint.

Blood sugar levels reflect your body's narrative—the silent stories swirling within your bloodstream. Regular checkups and tests become crucial chapters in your autobiography, revealing the peaks and valleys of your journey, and illuminating the path ahead.

Moreover, it's important to recognize the symbolic relationship between the body, the mind, and the communal aspects of life's banquet table. Blood sugar management connects deeply with this trinity, necessitating a balance that extends beyond the physical into the emotional and spiritual realms. Yes, insulin is a medication, a therapy, but it is also a symbol of the body's need for equilibrium, a signpost along your path to healing.

Take heart, for you are not Icarus flying solo towards the sun. Instead, you are amongst companions on a common voyage, each facing their storms, yet all journeying towards a destination of health and harmony. Your daily choices form the habits that, like threads in a loom, weave the majestic tapestry of your life story—a story destined for wholeness and youthful vitality, regardless of age.

As you press forward, remember that managing diabetes is like tending to a garden—it requires patience, dedication, and a gentle hand. It teaches you about the delicate balance of nature and nourishes your soul just as much as your body.

May your understanding of insulin and blood sugar not be merely intellectual, but a deeply rooted consciousness that empowers and liberates. The wisdom of the ages is your ally, and within it, you will find the strength to face each day with courage and grace, transforming challenges into victories, one step at a time.

Embrace this role of insulin and blood sugar with an open heart, for it is not just a biological process but a call to a higher standard of living—a summons to live fully, love deeply, and journey boldly towards the horizons of your life's potential. With every sunrise comes the promise of a new day, and with it, the opportunity to live well with diabetes. This is not the end of a chapter in your life but the beginning of a new, radiant narrative.

Risk Factors and Early Signs you've learned about the essence of type 2 diabetes and the central role of insulin and blood sugar in your body. Now, we turn our attention to unraveling the threads of risk and the whispers of early signs that herald the arrival of diabetes. Understanding these can be a beacon, guiding you toward proactive steps in safeguarding your well-being.

In the tapestry of risk factors, genetics plays a formidable role. If your family tree has roots tangled with diabetes, your vigilance should be keener. This does not decree your fate, but advises you of the need for mindful living - for our days are shaped more by our choices than by our genes. For me, my diagnosis came about at the same age as my father was when he was also diagnosed with diabetes.

Obesity is another clear clarion call, often an echo of modernity's sedentary chorus and abundant table. Excess weight, particularly around your midsection, can invite insulin resistance, the specter that looms over the onset of type 2 diabetes. But consider this not a sentence but a signal to embrace healthier habits.

Age, too, whispers its warnings; aging is inevitable, but it's also a canvas on which you paint your years with vibrancy or neglect. After forty-five, the risk of diabetes grows, a reminder that our temples of flesh require more diligent care as time carves its runes upon us.

Hypertension and high cholesterol are silent trumpeters, oft ignored until their call crescendos into dire straits. They hint at a cardiovascular system under duress, and their association with diabetes is a call to action to soothe these silent alarms with lifestyle changes.

For women, a history of gestational diabetes is a flag upon the field of health; it signals that your body has once danced to the erratic tune of blood sugar. Pay heed to these rhythms, and be ever watchful for their subtle return.

But risk factors are but half of the story. Early signs are the other, often so mild and unassuming they pass unnoticed among the rush of daily life. Frequent urination, a cascade that interrupts your slumber night after night, is an early whisper of sugar's overabundance in your bloodstream.

Thirst that seems unquenchable, the kind that no fountain can sate, speaks of your body's attempt to dilute this unwelcome sweet. Likewise, hunger that grows insatiable, gnawing at you despite a feast, hints at the inefficacy of glucose entering your cells. Heed these signs - they are missives urging you towards medical counsel.

Blurry vision might easily be dismissed as fatigue or age; yet, it too can be a signet of sugar's excess, a symbol that your body's delicate harmony is askew. Do not turn a blind eye, but rather, seek insight.

Unexpected weight loss, though often welcomed in the halls of vanity, can be an uninvited guest signaling that your body cannot harness the nourishment you offer it. It is a hollow victory, one that calls not for celebration but for examination.

Fatigue lays heavy upon many in this hurried life, but when rest no longer replenishes your vigor, it's time to ponder if a deeper drain is present. Persistent tiredness is not merely the result of life's toil but may whisper of the silent skirmish of diabetes within.

Slow-healing sores and frequent infections are the body's muted protests, a defense compromised, a fortress besieged. These aren't mere inconveniences, but signals from the ramparts that not all is well.

Tingling or numbness in your extremities, a sense of pins and needles where none should be, is like a watchman's bell, sounding the alarm that blood sugar's trespass has begun its work on your nerves. Heed these sensations; they guide you to seek sanctuary through medical attention.

These risk factors and early signs are not curses but opportunities; a chance to step into the light of awareness and act. Each one is like a thread in the hands of the Divine, reminding us we are woven together in a tapestry of cause and effect, personal responsibility and grace.

Embracing these warnings with a heart of courage and conviction can transform them from harbingers of distress to prophets of a healthier path. As you move forward, let these insights sculpt your journey toward a life not defined by diabetes, but informed and refined by the understanding and management of it.

It is of the utmost importance that we not only know, but educate those that we love on the early signs of diabetes. My personal journey with diabetes almost ended before I even realized that something was seriously wrong with my body. I was experiencing many of the classic signs, but didn't know at the time, that these were in fact, signs that my body was sending me that something was seriously wrong. By the time that I drug myself into the emergency room, I could barely function.

My A1C was over 11, my blood sugar was over 1100 and my bodies organs were in the early stages of giving up. I was quite literally in the early stages of dying. When I walked into the emergency room, they did a couple of test and admitted me in critical condition. I ended up having to stay there much longer than I would have liked.

And in this journey, remember to walk not in fear, but in faith. For it is often in facing our giants that we find our strength; in acknowledging our vulnerability, we discover our resilience; in confronting our challenges, we unearth our hope. Onward, then, with eyes open to the signs and steadfast in the belief that every day is a step toward balance and vitality.

Chapter 2:
Receiving the Diagnosis

The moment of receiving a type 2 diabetes diagnosis can feel like an abrupt interruption to the life you once knew, echoing a sense of trepidation amidst the unknowns that lie ahead. In the stillness of that doctor's office, your heart may have sunk as the weight of the words settled in, but let that moment be not the harbinger of despair but rather the beginning of a transformative journey. As the reality of your diagnosis unfolds, it's natural for a tumult of emotions to cascade through you—fear, denial, perhaps even guilt. Yet, within the fabric of these trying times, there's an opportunity to weave a tapestry of courage, hope, and renewal as you stand at the crossroads of a life altered, not ended. The path to managing diabetes is tread by taking one resolute step after another, starting with understanding the emotional whirlwind you're facing and gathering the fortitude to take those first, crucial steps towards well-being. Together, let's navigate through the uncertainty and move forward with unwavering determination, for you're not simply enduring a condition; you're embarking on a profound journey that will demand the best of who you aspire to be.

Handling the Emotions Discovering that one has been diagnosed with type 2 diabetes can trigger a cascade of emotions. It's a moment that may redefine how we see ourselves, our future, and our daily habits. For many, this news brings forth an initial tide of shock and denial. It's a natural human response to unexpected life changes, but it's essential to gradually move beyond these feelings to address the condition head-on.

Yet, as one takes time to process the diagnosis, it's not uncommon for fear to take hold. Questions about complications and necessary lifestyle adjustments can lead to a palpable sense of anxiety. However, remember, "For God has not given us a spirit of fear, but of power and of love and of a sound mind" (2 Timothy 1:7). There's strength within you, kindled by divine love and wisdom, to navigate this journey.

Anger and frustration may also arise. One might ask, "Why me?" or lament the perceived unfairness of the situation. It's valuable to acknowledge and express these emotions rather than suppress them, while also recognizing that they are transitory feelings on the path to acceptance and action.

Bargaining may follow, where you might find yourself making promises or commitments in hopes of reversing the diagnosis. While such deals with oneself may not change the diagnosis, they can be transformed into motivation for implementing healthier lifestyle choices, turning the bargaining into a bridge towards positive change.

Depression is another emotional layer that might envelop you. You may feel overwhelmed by the demands of managing diabetes or grieve for the loss of a previous, carefree way of life. Yet, it's written, "Cast all your anxiety on Him because He cares for you" (1 Peter 5:7). Sharing your struggles with a Higher Power can bring solace and strength when the weight seems too heavy to bear alone.

Ultimately, acceptance paves the way to empowerment. Embracing your diagnosis as a part of your life story, rather than a final summation of your health, can liberate you to make informed, proactive decisions. With a spirit of acceptance, you can foster resilience and a proactive mindset towards your diabetes management.

Transforming fear into courage is an essential aspect of your emotional journey. Reflecting on the scripture, "I can do all this through Him who gives me strength" (Philippians 4:13), can fortify your resolve to overcome the daily challenges of living with diabetes. Recognizing your strength can steer you toward the latter stages of emotional healing, where fear gives way to bravery and resolve.

Guilt, too, may surface if one believes that their actions or lifestyle contributed to the development of diabetes. Shedding this guilt is vital, as it serves no productive purpose. Understanding that diabetes can result from a complex interplay of genetics and environment can help ease these self-accusations.

Allowing oneself the grace to feel every emotion without judgment is an integral step in the healing process. As it says in Ecclesiastes, "There is a time for everything, and a season for every activity under the heavens" (Ecclesiastes 3:1). Each emotion plays a role in the grand tapestry of our experiences and enables growth and greater understanding.

Hope is a powerful emotion that can light the way through darker times. Looking ahead at the advancements in diabetes care, the testimonials of those who've soared beyond the challenges, and the promise of ongoing support can kindle a flame of optimism in your heart.

It's also vital to acknowledge the need for professional assistance when handling these emotions. Counseling or therapy, particularly with specialists familiar with chronic disease management, can provide valuable coping strategies and new perspectives to aid in emotional healing.

Finding solace in community and shared experiences can also buffer the emotional rollercoaster. Support groups offer spaces to voice concerns, share victories, and receive encouragement from those who truly understand the nuances of living with diabetes.

Throughout every emotional high and low, maintain a sense of patience with yourself. Managing diabetes is a lifelong process, and coming to terms with the emotional aspects of the disease does not happen overnight. Being kind to oneself and embracing the gift of patience can make the journey more manageable and more meaningful.

Being proactive in your emotional health will, in turn, positively impact your physical health. Just as managing your diet and exercise is crucial in diabetes care, so too is monitoring and nurturing your emotional well-being.

Finally, knowing that you're not on this path alone can make an immeasurable difference. Whether it be through the comfort of family, the wisdom of a higher power, or the camaraderie of the diabetes community, there's a multifaceted support system available to you. Each step you take, each emotion you experience, is part of a greater journey towards health and enlightenment.

First Steps After Diagnosis As the light streams through the window marking a new dawn, so too does your journey with diabetes begin anew. Receiving a Type 2 diagnosis might feel like a tempest has shaken your world. But, consider this moment not as a tempest but as an awakening, a call to elevate your life through understanding, transformation, and hope.

In the cool quiet of this genesis, it is crucial to remember that life does not end with this news—it flourishes in the presence of courage and deliberate action. Your first step on this path is gathering knowledge, for it is written, "My people are destroyed for lack of knowledge" (Hosea 4:6). Seek to understand the mechanisms of diabetes, how it affects your temple—the body—and what it means for your future. This understanding lays the foundation for all the actions and decisions that will follow.

Next, you are to grasp the significance of the numbers; your blood sugar levels will become indicators of your body's balance. As you monitor your glucose, think of it not as a judgment, but as a marker, much like a lighthouse guiding ships to port, allowing you to navigate the wellness of your body.

Then, you must cultivate a garden of support, planted firmly in the soil of community, friendship, and medical counsel. Establish connections with healthcare providers who are not merely professionals, but partners in your journey. Unearth local or digital support groups, where shared stories become the balm for the inevitable moments of distress.

Concomitantly, step into the practice of reflective journaling or prayer. In words or silence, find the strength of the psalmist who authored countless laments, celebrations, and prayers from the depths of human experience. Let your thoughts and feelings in the wake of diagnosis be known, be felt, and be offered up.

Embrace the art of nourishment, not merely as a matter of dietary restriction but as culinary discovery. Before delving into specifics of diabetic diets, which will unfold in due time, commit to a philosophy of balance, generosity, and intention with the food you consume.

Furthermore, consider physical activity not as a rigorous commandment but as a celebration of movement. Whether it is a gentle walk in the park or a harmonious yoga session, each step, each stretch is a victory in the campaign for your well-being.

Preparation is also a key ally. Assemble a diabetes care kit that includes a glucose meter, test strips, and emergency snacks. Prepare your habitat, your spaces of living and work, with mindful corners for rest and reflection, for both are as critical as the air you breathe.

What's more, there is wisdom in arranging your affairs, attending to the logistics of life with diabetes. Become acquainted with your medical insurance, knowing well the provisions and support it offers. Verify that your access to required medications and supplies is secured, as they are both your shield and your staff in this journey.

Sow seeds of dialogue with your loved ones, sprouting an environment where misunderstanding and fear can be uprooted. Educate them, gently and firmly, about your condition, transforming ignorance into a shared language of support and empathy.

And while you're at it, remember to savor the small victories and the everyday accomplishments. Every wise choice, every positive step, is a glimmering stone in the mosaic of your triumph over diabetes. Celebrate the good days and be gentle with yourself during the ones that challenge your resolve.

Amidst all these steps, arm yourself with patience. Though the world clamors for instantaneous cures and quick fixes, the path of managing diabetes is a testament to patient, persistent change and daily dedication. As the Scripture says, "But they that wait upon the Lord shall renew their strength" (Isaiah 40:31). Thus, wait upon the renewed strength that will burgeon from within as you walk this path.

Commit to learning continuously, for the world of diabetes care is ever-evolving. Stay abreast of the latest trends in treatment, not as a passive observer but an active participant in shaping your destiny. Seek out reputable resources that will fill your quiver with the arrows of knowledge.

Last but not least, these first steps culminate in a promise—a promise to yourself. This vow is a tapestry of grace, woven with the threads of self-compassion, understanding, and resolve. Recognize that this is not a journey towards perfection but progress, not an expedition marred by fear, but an odyssey empowered by grace and grit.

As we journey through later chapters tackling diet specifics, exercise formulations, and mental health strategies, let these initial steps be your bedrock. May they ground you in unwavering resolve as the next chapters of your life not only unfold but flourish, with you as the dignified author of your narrative, your Odyssey with diabetes.

Building Your Support Team As you step forward on your journey with diabetes, one thing becomes crystal clear: no one should have to walk this path alone. Throughout the scripture, we see the importance of fellowship, community, and bearing one another's burdens. In living with Type 2 diabetes, these principles hold profound significance; constructing a robust support team can be a wellspring of strength, comfort, and practical assistance.

First, recognize the multidimensional spectrum of "support." This isn't merely about having someone to remind you of your medication. It's discovering those special individuals who bring different flavors of encouragement, insight, and aid to your life. A variety of helping hands can mold what might feel like a colossal challenge into a manageable part of your daily routine.

Primary in your network is your healthcare team, a beacon highlighting your path. This group should include your primary care physician, a certified diabetes educator, an endocrinologist specialized in hormonal imbalances, and perhaps a dietitian. Their expertise is the cornerstone of your care, grounded in medical science and committed to your wellness journey.

Yet, the sinews connecting the bones of medical advice are found in your personal relationships. Family and friends can be just like Simon of Cyrene for you, helping to carry your cross when the burden gets heavy. They can be the ones you turn to, not only for practicalities like attending appointments but also for emotional sustenance on trying days.

Moreover, explore support groups, either locally or online. Just as the early church gathered in unity, these communities provide an opportunity to break bread with those who truly understand your experience with diabetes. In these circles, you can speak freely and learn from others facing similar trials and victories.

Faith can be a sanctuary, and spiritual guidance plays a pivotal role for many. Whether it's your pastor, rabbi, imam, or another spiritual leader, they can offer another dimension of support. Through prayer, wisdom, and spiritual counsel, they can lead you to find peace and strength that transcends the physical aspect of your condition.

Do not forget the role of neighbors and colleagues. They might not share your personal life, yet their daily presence and understanding can alleviate stress in your work and social environment. Openness about your condition, as much as you are comfortable with, can foster accommodations that make day-to-day efforts less taxing.

Professional counseling should never be undermined. Like the skilled craftsmen in biblical times who helped build the temple, counselors have the tools to help you construct a healthy mindset. They can guide you through the emotional labyrinth that often accompanies chronic illness and lead you to higher ground of emotional well-being.

Alongside these human pillars of support, consider the assistance of technology. Apps and devices can be like the star leading the Magi—guiding your way in monitoring blood sugar, meal planning, or even providing reminders for medication. Embrace these digital allies as part of your support network.

Remember, your support team isn't static; it's a living, breathing entity that should evolve as your needs change. Periodically assess and adjust your circle of support. Like seasons, some people or services may come and go, and that's okay. It's all part of refining what works best for your journey.

Advocacy groups are also invaluable team members; they not only fight for your needs on a broader stage, but also offer a wealth of knowledge and resources. They can be a source of empowerment and a reminder that your voice matters in the fight against diabetes.

As surely as day follows night, there will come times of discouragement, even despair. It's in these darkest valleys that your support team becomes critical. Like Moses, who needed Aaron and Hur to hold up his arms, your team will undergird you, giving you strength to continue when your own might fail.

Build trust and communicate openly with your team. Similar to the relationship between David and Jonathan, trust is key to support and emotional safety. Open lines of communication create an environment where you feel free to share your struggles and triumphs, as well as your fears and hopes.

Lastly, do not underestimate the power of gratitude. As you give thanks for the help and support you receive, you reinforce the bond with your team and affirm the value of each member. A grateful heart not only enlightens your own spirit but also brightens the path of those who journey with you.

In conclusion, your support team is paramount in navigating the waters of life with diabetes. A blend of professional guidance, personal relationships, community support, spiritual direction, and digital tools shapes a tapestry of support as unique as you are. They are the hands that hold yours, the hearts that empower you, and the voices that encourage you to press on towards a life of fulfillment and purpose despite the storm of diabetes.

Chapter 3:
Crafting Your Nutritional Blueprint

As we close the chapter on understanding the initial steps after your diagnosis, we turn our attention to constructing a solid framework for your daily sustenance. A diabetes-friendly diet isn't just about avoidance; it's a celebration of the diverse array of foods that not only nourish your body but also stabilize your blood sugar and invigorate your spirit. Like a seasoned architect drafting a masterful plan, you'll learn to balance the delicate intricacies of carbohydrates, fibers, proteins, and fats—each a foundational block in your temple of health. Remember the proverb "Man does not live by bread alone," and so you shall discern how a wholesome diet, rich in nature's bounty, becomes your scripture for wellbeing. Charting the meals that feed your body's needs without spiking your sugar levels is a skill that becomes second nature with practice. In this chapter, we delve into the art and science of this blueprint, guiding you in recognizing the wealth of choices that await your loving preparation, and setting the table for a future where every bite is an act of self-care. The main goal is to know that eating with diabetes isn't a lifelong sentence to bland boring meals.

The Basics of a Diabetes-Friendly Diet As we journey forward into the lands of nourishment with the guidance of our renewed understanding, let us illuminate the path towards a diet that befriends the body challenged by type 2 diabetes. As if manna from heaven, the right foods can be both a comfort and a catalyst for improved health, turning the daily bread into a testament of care for one's temple.

Nourishment, that sacred sustainer of life, when chosen with wisdom, can transform your daily meals into a symphony of balance and wellness. A diabetes-friendly diet isn't a punitive measure, but rather an opportunity to embrace food as a source of life-sustaining energy. Begin with the cornerstone of such a path: whole, unprocessed foods, which are the beacons that light the way to a harmonious relationship with your body's needs.

Imagine your plate as a canvas, painted with vibrant vegetables, each color representing not just an aesthetic delight, but a bounty of essential vitamins and minerals. Green leafy vegetables, bright bell peppers, and deep purple eggplants – these are not just ingredients, but tools to manage your blood sugar levels and nourish your body's systems.

Fruits, those natural sweets gifted to us from trees and vines, are to be enjoyed with consideration. While they are wholesome, their natural sugars remind us of the importance of balance and portion control. Integrate fruits with a mindful approach, focusing on fiber-rich choices like berries and apples, which offer their sweetness alongside a garden of nutrients, without causing rapid spikes in blood sugar.

Amidst this bounty, one must also consider lean proteins, the building blocks of repair and strength in the body. Fish that swim the depths of the sea, poultry grazing the fields, and legumes grown in the earth's embrace, all contribute to a robust and diverse diet. Proteins provide not only the means to rebuild but also the satisfaction of a meal that can satiate and sustain one's energy throughout the day.

As we speak of satiety, let us not forget the humble yet mighty grain – whole, intact, and brimming with nutrients. Grains like quinoa, barley, and oats can be likened to the grains of sand in an hourglass, slowly releasing energy as time wears on, avoiding the sudden tide of sugar that more refined grains might release into the bloodstream.

Hydration — the river of life that flows within us must never run dry. Water, unsweetened teas, and other non-caloric beverages help maintain the hydration so vital for all bodily functions. Like a well from which we can draw endlessly, without adding the weight of unnecessary sugars to our system.

Equally important is the art of restraint, for there is wisdom in moderating foods high in added sugars and saturated fats. As the ancient proverb teaches, "To everything, there is a season," — a time for every indulgence under heaven, but in moments sparing and sparse. These foods, while permissible on occasion, should not form the foundation of your temple's sustenance.

In the bread of affliction, there is understanding, and it's crucial to acknowledge that processed foods and fast food may offer convenience but at a significant cost to one's blood sugar stability. Opt instead for the effort of preparation, for even the simplest meal, crafted by your own hands, carries the imprint of intention and care.

Portion sizes, in their measured grace, serve to remind us that our bodies require only what is necessary for sustenance, not excess. Each meal is an opportunity to reflect on the provision and to consume not out of abundance, but out of need, respecting the body's signals of fullness and satisfaction.

Understanding the glycemic index and the load each food imparts upon your blood can become a daily meditation, a reflection upon the effects of sustenance upon your wellbeing. Choose foods with low to moderate glycemic values to maintain the gentle ebb and flow of sugars, rather than the tumultuous waves that higher glycemic foods may unleash.

As you make these dietary considerations, be mindful not to walk this path alone. In the assembly of diverse food choices lies the strength of your diet. Like the many members of a body, each food group contributes its function for the well-being of the whole. It's a balance, a harmony that one must strive for with every meal.

Let us also remember the value of joy in eating. The breaking of bread is a communal act, a ritual that brings together not only the body and spirit but also the company of loved ones. Let your meals be a time of fellowship and gratitude, embracing the pleasures of taste and the nourishment of companionship.

Lastly, do not be disheartened by the occasional divergence from the path. There is forgiveness in this journey, and every moment is a new chance to embrace the principles that protect and sustain life. With every new sunrise, we are presented with a fresh possibility to make choices that honor our health.

The basics of a diabetes-friendly diet are found not only in the food consumed but also in the spirit in which it is eaten. Embrace each meal with mindfulness, and let each bite be a testament to a life cherished and a body revered. For in the wisdom of nourishment lies the secret to a life lived abundantly with type 2 diabetes.

Reading and Understanding Food Labels is an essential skill that serves as a beacon, guiding you through the abundant choices in the grocery store while managing type 2 diabetes. Imagine walking down an aisle, an array of colors and options on either side, and knowing that you possess the knowledge to discern which items align with your health goals. This empowers you to make wise decisions that can improve your control over diabetes and promote overall well-being.

Firstly, let's consider the nutritional facts label found on packaged foods, which is designed to inform you about the contents of what you're about to consume. Understanding this information is akin to understanding a profound truth that sets you free to make educated choices. At the top of this label, you'll find serving size and servings per container. This speaks volumes; it's crucial to recognize that the nutritional values listed are often for a single serving, not the entire package.

The next critical aspect is the number of total carbohydrates, which includes starches, fiber, sugar, and sugar alcohols. In managing type 2 diabetes, carbs have a direct impact on blood sugar levels. Therefore, seek out the wisdom in these numbers as if they were a source of life. Remember, not all carbs are created equal—the fiber content, for instance, is beneficial because it has limited effect on blood sugar and can aid in digestion.

Sugars, both natural and added, are also illuminated on the label. Discerning the difference between these is crucial. The scriptures teach us that wisdom is more precious than rubies, and in this context, understanding the nuanced impact of naturally occurring sugars versus added sugars can be just as invaluable.

Protein content on the label should not be overlooked. Protein is an important ally in blood sugar regulation; it helps slow digestion and can lead to a more gradual rise in blood glucose levels. Just as the body needs strength, your diet needs the stability that protein offers.

Pay close attention to the dietary fiber content. Like a tree planted by streams of water, which yields its fruit in season, a diet rich in fiber can help you feel full longer and can have a positive effect on blood sugar levels. Fiber is also known for its role in heart health, which is particularly important for individuals with diabetes.

Fats, including saturated and trans fats, are also listed on the label. These should be approached with caution and wisdom, remembering that the body is a temple and must be treated with respect. Opt for foods low in unhealthy fats, which can increase the risk of heart disease.

Sodium content is another important factor, especially since high blood pressure is a common companion to diabetes. Like a city with walls, a well-guarded diet limits excessive sodium to protect the heart from assault.

Vitamins and minerals, though often listed at the very bottom, are not to be underestimated. They can be seen as the reinforcements that support the body's diverse functions, like warriors skilled in combat, enhancing overall health.

Ingredients lists are equally telling but are frequented less often by hurried shoppers. However, this list holds the truth of what you're truly consuming. Foods are listed in order of predominance, with the most prevalent ingredients first. Seek understanding here as if you were searching for hidden treasure, for within this list lies the reality of what the package contains.

Another tool at your disposal is the Percent Daily Value (%DV). This guide helps you understand the nutrients in the context of a total daily diet. While these percentages are based on a 2,000-calorie diet, you may require more or less depending on individual needs, but it still serves as a general framework for comparison.

"Light," "low-fat," and "reduced sugar" are compelling terms, but they can be deceptive. A product that is light in one area may compensate with undesirable ingredients in another. The discerning eye is crucial; scrutiny can reveal if an alternative is truly better or simply cloaked in appealing language.

It's not only about the avoidance of certain ingredients; it's also about seeking out quality foods that nourish and sustain. Whole, unprocessed foods may not always come with labels, but they are often the most beneficial. Just as a house built on a solid foundation will stand, a diet based on whole foods will support long-term health.

Lastly, keep in mind that understanding food labels is an ongoing process. Food manufacturers often change their recipes or update labels. Therefore, vigilance and continual learning are your allies. Much like a journey of a thousand miles begins with a single step, so too does the mastery of food label literacy commence with reading the first label with intention.

As you embrace this knowledge and apply it to your grocery shopping, you will find strength in the choices you make. With each label you read and understand, you construct your health, choice by choice, as if laying down bricks to a well-fortified fortress. And from this place of strength, managing type 2 diabetes becomes less of a challenge and more of an achievable, daily practice.

In essence, reading and understanding food labels is not just about making smarter food choices, but it's about building a life more in line with the serenity of control and the joy of good health. As you navigate through your dietary choices, remember that the greatest wealth is health, and that wealth is well within your grasp. Stand firm in this knowledge, and let it be the lamp unto your feet, guiding you on this path of well-being.

Meal Planning and Prepping Strategies As we've explored the basics of a diabetes-friendly diet and how to navigate food labels, let's delve into a cornerstone practice for maintaining this lifestyle: meal planning and prepping. Having a clear plan for your meals can not only help regulate blood sugar levels but also reduce daily decision fatigue and keep you steadfast on your journey to better health.

Firstly, understand that your meals should have a balance of nutrients, with a particular focus on fiber-rich carbohydrates, lean proteins, and healthy fats. This balance is essential to maintaining energy levels and managing blood sugar. Consider the biblical principle of moderation and apply it to how you approach meal composition—you don't have to forsake all grains or indulge in every salad; it's about finding a balance that works for your body and spirit.

Start by mapping out a week's menu. Think of meals you enjoy that align with your dietary needs, and begin to sketch out a plan. Remember, it's not about perfection but progress. As it's said, 'Man does not live on bread alone,' and this holds especially true when man must consider his glycemic index. Broaden your palate with whole foods that not only satisfy but also nourish.

Once your menu is set, create a shopping list. This list should align with your meal plan, ensuring that you have all necessary ingredients without yielding to the temptations that can often arise when wandering the aisles without guidance. Just as a wise builder counts the cost before building, so you must plan before purchasing.

Prepping food can be a task that requires time and patience. Set aside a block of time each week for this purpose. Washing, chopping, and portioning out ingredients for the week ahead can be a meditative and reflective time. In life, as in food preparation, 'there is a time for everything', and the discipline of setting aside time to prepare will reap benefits throughout the week.

Consider cooking meals in larger batches. Whether through the use of a slow cooker, oven, or grill, creating larger portions can save you time and effort. Having ready-to-eat meals or meal components in your fridge or freezer makes it easier to stay within the boundaries of your nutritional blueprint when hunger strikes.

Labeling and dating your prepped meals and ingredients can be a helpful strategy. As with the parable of the talents, you've been entrusted with resources—investing a little time in organizing your fridge can cause your efforts to multiply, offering peace of mind and clarity when choosing your meals each day.

Adhering strictly to your meal plan isn't necessary—there's room for grace and flexibility in your diet, as there is in life. When special occasions or the unpredictable nature of life interfere, it's essential to adapt while still aiming for choices that align with your nutritional goals. Prioritize your health but remain adaptable, for 'to everything there is a season, and a time to every purpose.'

Equip yourself with the right tools—quality containers, a sharp set of knives, a reliable blender, or a food processor can all make meal prep more efficient and enjoyable. Just as David selected five smooth stones before facing Goliath, so too must you prepare your kitchen for success.

Record your blood sugar responses to different meals. By monitoring and understanding how your body reacts to certain foods, you refine your meal plan to better suit your unique needs. This self-awareness and personal data collection are invaluable for long-term management.

Invite family or friends to join you in the meal planning and prepping process. Not only can this be a time for fellowship, but it also helps those around you understand your needs and the importance of your dietary choices. 'Two are better than one; because they have a good reward for their labor.' Your journey is one shared with loved ones, each playing a role in your management of diabetes.

Stay hydrated. Often overlooked in meal prep is the role of fluids. Ensure you have easy access to water and avoid sugary drinks that can disrupt blood sugar levels. Just as the body craves water, so does your body need adequate hydration to optimally metabolize nutrients and maintain health.

Are you struggling for inspiration? Look to diabetes-friendly cookbooks or the abundance of digital resources available. New recipes can bring excitement to your palate and motivation to your spirit. Just as 'iron sharpens iron,' exploring and learning from others can enhance your culinary skills and your dietary regimen.

Finally, be kind to yourself. There may be days when things do not go as planned—a hastily chosen meal here or a missed prep session there. It's essential to remember that 'there is now no condemnation for those who are in Christ Jesus.' Do not be disheartened but resolve to start afresh with the next meal or the next day.

As you practice these meal planning and prepping strategies, you'll notice a transformation not merely in your physical health but also in your mental and spiritual well-being. There's a rhythm and a discipline to this practice that echoes the beauty found in many of life's journeys. With each step, you're not just crafting meals, but shaping a lifestyle that honours your body, emboldens your spirit, and enriches your life living with diabetes.

Chapter 4:
The Power of Exercise

As we forge ahead on this path of resilience and mindful living, it is paramount that we ignite a discussion on the profound influence of physical activity. Exercise, a cornerstone of well-being, has a transformative impact on those wrestling with type 2 diabetes. It transcends the simple act of movement and evolves into a powerful ally, enhancing insulin sensitivity and ushering in a balance of blood sugars that mirrors the harmony we seek in our daily lives. In the throes of exertion, one finds a quiet fortitude, a testament to the enduring spirit that defines our human experience.

Embracing exercise as a daily pillar is not merely about relentless pursuits but finding a rhythm that resonates with the body's needs and the soul's yearnings. In its essence, movement is a celebration of capability, a reminder that we are fearfully and wonderfully made, capable of overcoming the inertia that illness can impose. As we dedicate ourselves to this chapter in our lives, let us look upon exercise not as a daunting task but as a liberation, a reclaiming of the strength that flows through us, as indomitable as the currents of life itself.

Types of Exercise Beneficial for Type 2 Diabetes Moving from understanding and accepting a diabetes diagnosis to actively engaging in a lifestyle that supports your well-being is no small feat. As we step into the realm of physical activity, we understand that exercise is a cornerstone of diabetes management. For individuals with type 2 diabetes, specific forms of exercise can be particularly beneficial in controlling blood sugar levels and improving overall health.

One of the most foundational types of exercise is aerobic exercise. Also known as cardio, this form of activity elevates your heart rate and boosts your breathing. Examples include brisk walking, jogging, swimming, and cycling. These activities are known to increase insulin sensitivity and help your muscles use glucose more effectively. Aim for at least 150 minutes of moderate aerobic exercise spread throughout the week, remembering to start slowly and gradually intensify your activities as you gain strength and endurance.

Strength training is another critical component for diabetes care. By building muscle mass, you're not only sculpting your body but also creating more 'storage space' for glucose. Resistance exercises like weightlifting, using resistance bands, or bodyweight workouts such as push-ups and squats should be included in your routine at least twice a week. Don't be intimidated by the thought of heavy weights or packed gyms; strength training can be as straightforward as lifting canned goods at home or engaging in gardening tasks that require some muscle work.

Flexibility exercises should not be overlooked. Stretching, yoga, and Pilates can improve your range of motion, reduce stress, and aid in preventing injury. For someone living with diabetes, stress management is crucial as stress can affect blood sugar levels. Embrace these gentler forms of exercise to find balance and enhance your sense of peace, complementing the more intense elements of your fitness plan.

Balance exercises are especially vital for older adults with type 2 diabetes who may be at risk of falls. Practices such as Tai Chi or simple activities like standing on one foot can help improve your balance and coordination, all the while contributing to your overall fitness.

Now, it's important to note that exercise should not be a punishment; it is a celebration of what your body can do. Start with what you enjoy, be it dancing, gardening, or walking the dog, and let those activities be the foundation upon which you build a more structured plan. Engaging in physical activities you enjoy increases the likelihood that you'll stick with them long term.

High-intensity interval training (HIIT) might sound daunting, but it's been shown to be highly effective for people with type 2 diabetes. This type of training alternates between short bursts of intense exercise and periods of rest or lower-intensity exercise. The beauty of HIIT lies in its flexibility – you can tailor your intervals and exercises to your fitness level, and it can be incorporated into many different types of physical activity, such as running, biking, or rowing.

Remember, when it comes to exercise, consistency is key. It's not necessary to embark on strenuous workouts daily to observe a significant impact on your diabetes management. Instead, focus on developing a routine that is sustainable and enjoyable.

Furthermore, understand that each day holds potential for new beginnings. If you miss a workout or don't meet your exercise goals for the week, show yourself grace. Reflect on the words of Saint Paul in Philippians 4:13, "I can do all things through Christ who strengthens me." This passage is a powerful reminder that your strength and your capacity for change come not from within, but from above.

For those who might feel overwhelmed with structured workouts, incorporating physical activity into daily life can also make a significant difference. Taking the stairs instead of the elevator, parking further away from store entrances, or engaging in active play with your children or grandchildren can increase your activity level without the need for a gym membership or fitness equipment.

In the Garden of Eden, Adam was tasked with tending to the land – a form of physical labor that kept him active. Let this biblical principle guide you to view every chore or errand as an opportunity to care for your temple, your body, with the diligence it deserves.

It's essential to communicate with your healthcare provider before beginning any new exercise regimen, ensuring that the activities you choose align with your current health status and diabetes management plan.

In the wake of your diagnosis, keep in mind that exercise should not be a lone endeavor. Ecclesiastes 4:12 says, "Though one may be overpowered, two can defend themselves. A cord of three strands is not quickly broken." Build a support network that includes exercise partners, fitness professionals knowledgeable in diabetes care, or even a community group with similar health goals. These relationships can provide the encouragement and accountability necessary to make lasting lifestyle changes.

The path to diabetes management through exercise can also be seen as a pilgrimage; a journey that involves travel through various terrains, each with its own challenges and lessons. Embrace the journey with the knowledge that the road to better health is paved with persistence and small, continuous steps.

As you forge ahead, consider keeping an exercise log or journal as a way to track your progress, celebrate your victories, and address any challenges that arise. An exercise log can be a powerful motivational tool, revealing the true measure of the strides you've made over time.

In the realm of physical activity and diabetes management, there lies both challenge and opportunity. Embrace these various activities as your shields and weapons in the fight against type 2 diabetes, keeping in mind that your efforts today are an investment in a healthier tomorrow.

Creating a Sustainable Workout Routine As we have explored the importance of nutrition in managing type 2 diabetes, let us turn our focus to the other cornerstone of diabetes care—exercise. Knowing the types of exercises that can benefit you is just the beginning. The challenge, and the solution, lies in crafting a workout routine that is durable and resilient, one that stands the test of time and becomes a pillar of your lifestyle.

The scriptures guide us to understand that our body is a temple, and as such, it deserves care and respect. In creating a routine that honors our physical form, we must approach exercise not as a transient hobby but as a dedicated practice.

To start, consider your current level of fitness and how it intertwines with your diabetes management. You can't build a house without a foundation, so it's crucial to establish a baseline—a safe starting point from which to grow. Consult with your healthcare provider about any limitations or precautions before commencing or changing your routine.

Next, it's imperative to set realistic and achievable goals. As the adage goes, "Do not despise these small beginnings, for the Lord rejoices to see the work begin." Small, consistent steps lead to substantial progress. Whether it's a daily 15-minute walk or a twice-weekly swim, define what you can manage now, keeping in mind the flexibility to evolve as your fitness improves.

Diversity in your workout routine prevents monotony and can keep your motivation soaring. Include a mix of cardiovascular exercises, strength training, flexibility, and balance activities. Each type has unique benefits for diabetes management, such as improving insulin sensitivity and aiding in weight control.

Remember, discipline is the bridge between goals and accomplishment. Schedule your workouts as you would any important appointment. This commitment cements them into your routine and elevates their priority. An early morning session or an evening walk after dinner can integrate seamlessly into your life when consistently planned.

Adaptability is also critical. Just as there are seasons in nature, your exercise routine will have its own ebb and flow. There may be days when you feel weaker or your blood sugar levels aren't stable enough for your usual workout. Listen to your body's signals and be willing to adjust your plans accordingly.

To ensure sustainability, your workout routine should be enjoyable. Take pleasure in the movement of your body and the vitality it brings. Find activities that delight and engage you, whether it be dancing, gardening, or perhaps cycling. Make exercise a celebration of life rather than a chore.

Accountability can serve as a powerful motivator. Sharing your exercise journey with a friend or a group can bolster your commitment. Ecclesiastes reminds us that two are better than one, for they have a good return for their labor; use this wisdom to stay motivated and encouraged.

Tracking your progress is another way to maintain a sustainable routine. Use a journal or an app to note the exercises you've done, how you felt, and any changes in your blood sugar levels. This will not only document your journey but also help identify what works best for you. "For where there is no vision, the people perish." Let your records be your vision and keep you from perishing in enthusiasm.

Rest is not idleness, and sometimes doing nothing is as important as doing something. Rest days are crucial for recovery, allowing muscles to repair and grow stronger. Integrate rest into your regimen, honoring it as you would your most vigorous workout.

Lastly, patience and grace for yourself are vital as you embark on this healthier path. There will be setbacks and days when you fall short of your planned activities. Accept these without harsh judgment. Remember, "My grace is sufficient for you, for my power is made perfect in weakness." Allow yourself the grace to stumble and the strength to rise again.

A sustainable workout routine is a journey, not a destination. It should evolve as you do, flexing and adapting to your life's rhythm. With each step, each lift, and each stretch, you are not just moving your body; you are nurturing your temple and creating a harmony that resonates with self-care and self-respect.

As you develop this routine, remember to regularly consult with your healthcare team and revise it based on changes in your diabetes management. Work closely with your diabetes educator or physical therapist to modify exercises as needed to keep them safe and effective.

Let the wisdom from the ancients inspire you: "Physical training is of some value, but godliness has value for all things, holding promise for both the present life and the life to come." Your health is a gift, and cultivating a sustainable workout routine is one way to cherish this precious offering. Embrace it with the determination and hope that every new day brings.

Monitoring Your Blood Sugar During Activity is an essential aspect of managing type 2 diabetes that can be likened to a dance: a delicate balance of movement, rhythm, and awareness. As you integrate exercise into your life, it's crucial to understand that activity affects blood sugar levels in profound ways. Just as King David found strength and joy in movement, you too can discover the harmonious relationship between physical activity and your blood glucose control.

Remember the biblical account of the Israelites gathering manna, instructed to take only what they needed for the day? In a similar vein, monitoring your blood sugar provides immediate feedback about your current needs. Think of it as daily manna for your health, guiding you to the right amount of activity for your body's current state. Consistent monitoring helps you avoid the extremes of high and low blood sugar, which can be particularly troublesome during or after exercise.

The parable of building a house on a solid foundation applies well to the practice of monitoring: when you exercise, your muscles consume glucose at higher rates, and this can cause fluctuations. Like a wise builder, you need to measure these changes carefully to maintain the structure of good health. Sometimes, even a short walk can significantly impact your numbers, serving as a reminder that what seems small can be powerful.

It's important to note that different exercises have varied effects. While aerobic activities can lower your blood sugar during and immediately afterward, anaerobic exercises, such as weightlifting, may initially raise it. However, both types of activity increase insulin sensitivity overall, which is beneficial in the long term. This nuanced understanding can seem complex, but with time it becomes part of your wisdom, the discernment in balancing life with diabetes.

Timing is another critical element. Checking your blood sugar before exercise gives you a starting point: if it's low, you may need to eat a small snack to prevent hypoglycemia; if it's high, you might need to wait or adjust your insulin dose as advised by your healthcare provider. Just as each season has its purpose under heaven, each exercise session has its optimal timing in relation to your blood sugar levels.

While you're active, you also need to be vigilant. If you feel dizzy, shaky, or weak, test your blood sugar immediately. These could be signs that the lamp of your body needs refueling. On the other hand, remember that since the body and spirit are intertwined, sometimes what feels like a physical signal might be spiritual or emotional, and rest or reflection could be necessary.

After exercise, it's just as essential to monitor. You may experience delayed hypoglycemia up to several hours post-workout, so this vigilance can be seen as a watchman on the walls, ensuring that while your body rests, your blood sugar stays in safe ranges. It's not just about statistics; it's about protecting the temple of your body.

Moreover, documenting these numbers in a log serves as your personal scripture of health, a record of how your body responds to activity and the adjustments needed for optimal balance. In this way, you can learn from the past to better navigate the future, walking wisely in your journey with diabetes. Your journal becomes a testament of trials and victories, metrics that guide towards well-being.

Technological advancements also offer a helping hand, akin to the wisdom from above. Continuous glucose monitors (CGMs) can provide a more comprehensive picture of how exercise affects your blood sugar throughout the day, offering you a continuous stream of knowledge, much like the river of life that flows and sustains.

Adhering to a routine of monitoring also exercises your faith in the unseen. Though fluctuations in blood sugar may not always be immediate or evident, trusting in the process of regular checks and understanding the data can strengthen your commitment to self-care. Over time, your intuition becomes sharper, and you'll better anticipate how different activities influence your levels.

There will be days when blood sugar levels may not respond as anticipated, even with careful monitoring. Don't be discouraged, for every day has enough trouble of its own, but not without hope for tomorrow. Reflect on each experience and seek counsel if needed, knowing that each obstacle is an opportunity for growth and mastery over the condition.

A word of caution: While exercise is beneficial, it's important not to overburden the weary or overwork the body. Test frequently, adjust as necessary, and ensure that you're giving your body the restorative rest it needs. In the same way that the land was given a Sabbath for rest, so too should your body be allowed to recover.

In conclusion, monitoring your blood sugar during activity is a profound act of stewardship over the body you've been given. As you navigate this aspect of diabetes management, may you find the patience of a gardener tending to his crops, the steadiness of a shepherd watching his flock, and the joy of a dance that celebrates life in all its fullness.

With this foundation, you're now equipped to continue your journey with a vigilant heart. Embrace this practice as not just a medical necessity, but as a spiritual discipline that fosters mindfulness, responsibility, and a deeper connection with the rhythms of your body and life's unfolding path.

Chapter 5:
Medication and Monitoring

As the dawn ushers in a new day, so does knowledge empower us to take control of our health and well-being. In living with Type 2 diabetes, understanding the pivotal role of medication and meticulous blood glucose monitoring is akin to finding manna in the wilderness—it sustains and leads us to a healthier state. The wisdom contained in your treatment regimen is more than a routine—it's a testament to modern medicine's ability to emulate the body's natural rhythm of insulin production and blood sugar regulation. In this chapter, we invite you to delve into the harmonious dance between the medicines that help maintain your glycemic balance and the vigilant watch you keep over the ebb and flow of your blood sugar levels. It is here, in the pursuit of balance, that one finds the strength to not just endure, but to thrive amidst the challenges posed by diabetes. Indeed, within every dose of medication and each blood sugar reading, lies an opportunity for reflection, adjustment, and progress on your journey to wellness.

Common Medications for Type 2 Diabetes As we tread the path of understanding and managing type 2 diabetes, we recognize the value of a multipronged approach. Alongside the foundational pillars of diet and exercise, medications often play a crucial role in harmonizing the symphony of our body's functions. The landscape of medications for type 2 diabetes is broad, and knowing your options can empower you with knowledge and hope as you navigate this journey.

First, let us reflect on Metformin, a bastion of hope for many. It lowers glucose production in the liver, enhances insulin sensitivity, and helps usher glucose into the cells. This stalwart of diabetes treatment is a fortress for your blood sugar levels, helping to stave off the erratic spikes that can wreak havoc on your body.

Sulfonylureas, a class of medications that coax the pancreas into producing more insulin, are like the messengers that beckon a greater downpour of life-giving rains in a dry land. They can be effective, but must be taken with care, as they carry the risk of watering the land too much—leading to low blood sugar.

Contrarily, DPP-4 inhibitors are the gentle whisperers that tell the body to release insulin more slowly and thoughtfully, coordinating a response that is temperate and considerate of the body's intricate balance.

As we come upon SGLT2 inhibitors, we encounter a novel approach—urging the kidneys to excrete a portion of the glucose through urine. In this way, it's as if the body is guided to cast off excess baggage that could weigh down its voyage towards equilibrium.

We also discover GLP-1 receptor agonists, which are akin to a wise counselor advising restraint; they slow digestion and help curb the voracious appetite that often tempts one to stray from the path of moderation.

Thiazolidinediones, with their capability to increase insulin sensitivity, serve as builders, fortifying the cells' receptivity to insulin— a beacon of light in the efforts to assimilate nutrients with grace and ease.

Alpha-glucosidase inhibitors, while less commonly used, act as gatekeepers, slowing the breakdown of starches in the intestines. They remind us that sometimes slowing the pace can allow for a more measured and controlled absorption of life's sweetness.

Meglitinides can be likened to a call to action, prompting the body to release insulin in concordant waves with meals. Timing, as they demonstrate, can be everything when seeking to maintain balance.

And let us not forget insulin therapy itself—the cornerstone treatment for many, providing the very essence of what the body needs to utilize life's energy. The advent of insulin treatment reminds us of the promise of restoration, the possibility of replacing what is lacking, and restoring wholeness.

The world of diabetes medications is constantly evolving, so make sure to keep an open dialog with your medical support team. I have had to make some adjustments at times due to extended travel plans, shortages of certain medications etc.... Think of your medical support team like the pit crew of a professional racing driver. It is your job to let them know what is going on, and it is their job to make and execute a plan to fix it. You as the driver must take that plan and get out there and win the race.

In considering these medications, it's essential to understand that each person's journey is unique—what works for one may not work for another. Like a well-tended garden, the proper combination of tools, treatments, and care can create a flourishing environment conducive to health and vitality.

Moreover, just as wisdom is acquired through a lifetime of experiences, understanding which medication or combination of medications is most effective may take time and experimentation under the guidance of a healthcare provider.

Monitoring your progress will become a part of your daily rhythm, helping you identify how your body responds to these medications. In this, we see the parallel to the daily practice of reflection and growth—one that takes patience, commitment, and faith in the process.

Side effects are also part of the narrative when dealing with medications, reminding us that every action may have an opposite reaction. Open dialogue with your doctor and persistent testing ensure that your tailored regimen continues to serve your needs and well-being.

Affordability and access to medication may also present themselves as challenges along the way. But be encouraged, for there are many advocacy groups, assistance programs, and resources to support you on this expedition of managing your health.

Embrace each day with the knowledge that, while the battle may be arduous, the war can be won—with perseverance, support, and the right pharmacological allies, you can wield control over diabetes and live a life that is not only sustained but also enriched by the depth of your experience. For in every challenge, there is an opportunity to emerge stronger and more enlightened than before.

Mastering Blood Glucose Monitoring is like navigating through a dense forest where each tree represents a unique challenge or variable in your diabetes management journey. Blood glucose monitoring isn't just about getting a number; it's about understanding your body's intimate language and how it responds to different stimuli like food, stress, exercise, and medication. As someone living with diabetes, becoming adept at this can transform your daily life, offering clarity and control over a condition that can often feel unpredictable.

As you have ventured through crafting a nutritional blueprint and acknowledged the immense power of exercise, remember that these actions are intertwined with the need to monitor your blood glucose. To establish a strong foundation for managing your diabetes, you must first embrace the process of learning to track your blood sugar levels. This is not purely a scientific task; it is one of personal growth and self-awareness.

Consider the act of checking your blood glucose as an act of stewardship over the temple of your body, much as the biblical principle of stewardship teaches one to be responsible and diligent with what they have been entrusted. Monitoring becomes a focal point for taking ownership of your health. It's about being vigilant, like the watchmen of ancient walls, anticipating the early signs of fluctuation that could indicate a need to adjust your course.

To start, familiarize yourself with your meter. Spend time understanding its functions, quirks, and how to keep it properly calibrated. All of this is part of becoming proficient in gathering the data your body provides. Just as a diligent farmer knows the time to sow and the time to reap, you too will learn the right times to check and respond to your blood glucose levels.

"For everything there is a season, and a time for every matter under heaven." - This timeless wisdom from Ecclesiastes also applies to the realm of blood glucose monitoring. There are pivotal times to test: upon waking, before meals, two hours after meals, before exercise, and at bedtime. These specific times give you insight into how your body's glucose levels change throughout the day and night.

Create rituals and routines around your monitoring—like Daniel in the lion's den, let nothing shake your resolve to maintain these habits. Whether you face trials or feast in times of plenty, let regular monitoring be your unwavering practice. Through consistency comes the understanding and thus the ability to predict and manage your body's responses with greater accuracy.

Document your readings meticulously, just as one would chronicle a journey. This logbook becomes not just a recording but a repository of knowledge that can empower both you and your healthcare providers. Patterns revealed in this written account can guide adjustments in diet, exercise, and medication. It is written: "Write the vision; make it plain on tablets, so he may run who reads it."

Learning to interpret the numbers is akin to understanding a new language. Just as one would ponder a proverb, delve into what each glucose reading indicates. Feel empowered to adjust your meal plan if you notice consistent postprandial spikes, or to speak with your doctor about medication changes if your fasting glucose levels are not within the target range.

Don't walk alone on this path. Engage your healthcare team frequently and let them be like Aaron and Hur, supporting Moses' hands during battle. They can help elucidate the cryptic aspects of your results and provide professional insight. Proverbs tells us that in an abundance of counselors, there is victory—a principle that bears true in managing diabetes.

Embrace technology as a helpful ally in your quest. Continuous Glucose Monitors (CGMs) and insulin pumps can provide additional layers of data and support, offering a more dynamic picture of your glucose trends throughout the day. These devices, though intimidating at first, can become like the stones David chose from the brook—tools precisely picked for your battle against diabetes.

As you face challenges in mastering blood glucose monitoring, remember that each test, each note, is a step toward a more enlightened state of health. Each drop of blood holds a story that can guide you to better choices and brighter days. Let perseverance be your companion, knowing that patience produces character, and character produces hope. And hope does not put us to shame.

As the apostle Paul encouraged the Philippians to press on toward the goal, you also must press on in the daily management of your condition. Take time to celebrate the victories — no matter how small — as each successful reading is an affirmation of your diligent work and commitment.

Curiosity should also accompany you on this journey. Explore how different foods, exercises, and even stress levels affect your blood sugar. Your body is a temple uniquely yours, and understanding how it responds to various aspects of life can arm you with the wisdom to make informed decisions for better control.

Finally, understand that mastering blood glucose monitoring is a continuous journey and integral in the grander voyage of living fully with diabetes. As you aim to attain a holistic sense of well-being, let the words of the psalmist resonate: "Teach us to number our days that we may get a heart of wisdom." May this wisdom guide you to lead a life of balance, health, and vitality.

When to Adjust Your Treatment Plan As you walk this path of managing type 2 diabetes, remember that your journey is unique, and so is your treatment. Your relationship with your treatment plan is not static; it's a dynamic, ongoing conversation between you and your healthcare team, echoing the needs of your body and the rhythms of your life. There may be moments when adjustments are needed, times to reevaluate, and opportunities to refine your approach.

Consider the manifold seasons of life – just as each brings its own beauty, challenges may arise that necessitate change. If you're experiencing persistent blood sugar levels that are too high or too low despite your adherence to your current regimen, it's a clear signal to revisit your treatment strategy. Your body might be speaking, telling you that it's time to calibrate the tools and tactics in your arsenal.

Another hallmark moment inviting change is the onset of new symptoms or complications. A watchful eye on how your body is responding is crucial; vigilance leads to wisdom in making timely corrections. Be attentive to your body's whispers so they don't have to become shouts for you to listen.

Have you been blessed with the joyful news of weight loss that has been sustained over time? This significant achievement can also mean your body requires less medication to manage your diabetes. Reduction in weight often leads to better insulin sensitivity, an opportunity to decrease medication under your doctor's supervision.

Conversely, if you encounter an increase in weight, this too can impact your treatment plan. Weight can influence insulin resistance, possibly requiring a different approach to medication, diet, or exercise to maintain control of your glucose levels.

Furthermore, life isn't without its stresses – emotional upheavals or physical ones like illness or injury. These stressors can have formidable effects on blood sugar levels. Therefore, your treatment plan should be flexible enough to accommodate these times, ensuring stability amidst life's inevitable storms.

As you age, your treatment plan may require adjustments. Aging affects your body's insulin use and glucose production. It's a natural ebb and flow that calls for treatment alignment to ensure ongoing effectiveness and to avoid potential over- or under-treatment.

Should you find yourself blessed with access to new technology or medications, this too is an occasion to appraise your current plan. Proactive engagement with innovations can offer improved management tactics, enhanced convenience, and the potential for better outcomes.

There may be changes in your daily routines, perhaps a transition to a more active lifestyle or a shift in your dietary preferences or needs. Your treatment plan must be nimble, adaptable to the variances in how you live your daily life to help you maintain glycemic control.

Stay informed and conversant with your healthcare provider about the potential impacts of other medications you're prescribed for separate conditions. Interdependencies between drugs can influence your diabetes management, requiring an astute recalibration of your medication and monitoring strategy.

Pregnancy or planning for it entails profound body changes and necessitates a careful reevaluation of your treatment plan. Pondering the creation of life within, you must ensure your glucose levels are strictly managed to safeguard both your health and that of your unborn child.

Repeated hypoglycemic episodes, those deeply concerning low blood sugar events, are a signpost that you must alter your plan. Hypoglycemia can be dangerous, and avoiding its repeated instances can be as essential as managing high sugar levels – both require a balanced, disciplined approach.

If your regular tests and check-ups start exhibiting altered patterns, it's wise to understand the story they're narrating. These tools, these gifts of insight, allow us to detect subtle shifts that might otherwise go unnoticed, guiding us to make informed decisions about our care.

Moreover, the evolution of your goals can initiate changes to your treatment plan. Destiny is not a matter of chance; it's a matter of choice. If you set new health targets, your diabetes management regime should support your aspirations, acting as a bridge to your desired future.

In the face of these indicators for change, take heart and approach each adjustment not as a setback but as a step forward in the quest for balance and wellness. Reflect upon the wisdom of Proverbs: "A person's heart plans his way, but the Lord directs his steps." Embrace each adjustment, each directed step, as divine guidance, delivering you to a place of better health and greater understanding of your body's needs. It's an ongoing testament to the resilient spirit within you that perseveres and adapts in pursuit of a fulfilling life with diabetes.

Chapter 6:
The Weight Management Connection

As we have learned from our foundational knowledge of type 2 diabetes, the journey towards optimal health is indeed a tapestry woven with many threads, and among these is the critical element of weight management. 'The Weight Management Connection' is not solely about the numbers on a scale, but an opportunity for transformation, a chance to fine-tune the temple that is your body. For those living with diabetes, balancing the scales can mean enhancing insulin sensitivity, and scripturally, as our bodies are temples, it's our duty to steward them prudently. Knowing that your body is designed to thrive, managing weight becomes a profound act of worship, placing importance on the dietary choices made at the table as much as the psalms sung in the heart. It's in embracing the interplay of nourishment and movement that we find endeavors like weight loss are not merely tasks but expressions of a deeper commitment to health—a manifestation of the belief that through honoring the vessel given to us, we are engaging in a quiet dialogue of self-care and self-respect. This chapter is a robust lighthouse guiding you to the shore of understanding, as managing your weight is not just a chapter in your life, it's an ongoing narrative in the story of your well-being, filled with chapters of hope, perseverance, and renewal.

The Impact of Weight on Diabetes Control As we navigate through the fundamentals of managing type 2 diabetes, one topic of paramount significance emerges: the intricate link between weight and diabetes control. To understand this connection, we must look closely at how our body mass affects insulin resistance and blood sugar levels. Bear in mind, this isn't just about numbers on a scale; it's about the incredible journey your body undertakes to maintain harmony within.

Your weight carries a profound impact on how effectively you can manage diabetes. Excess body fat, especially around the waist, acts as a barrier to insulin's ability to work efficiently. This resistance forces the pancreas to work harder, producing more insulin in an effort to keep blood sugar levels in check. Over time, this can lead to what's known in medical terms as beta-cell burnout. Much like a well that runs dry, the pancreas might no longer keep up with the body's increased insulin demands.

Consider the parable of the sower. Just as seeds flourish in good soil, so too will your cells respond better to insulin without the obstacle of excess weight. Indeed, shedding even a modest amount of weight can result in significant improvements in insulin sensitivity. In this sense, managing your weight doesn't just lighten the physical load on your frame; it eases the burden on your cells.

It is important to remember that you are not alone in this struggle. Many face the mountain that is weight management, and it's okay to seek guidance. Maintaining a healthy weight is akin to finding balance, much like the scales of justice. It's about equitable measures—taking in just as much nourishment as your body requires, no more and no less.

Reducing your weight can also have a cascading effect on your overall health. Not only does it bolster diabetes control, but it also decreases the risk of cardiovascular diseases—akin to calming stormy seas. Your body is a temple, and as you respect its structures, you guard against the wear of winds and waters—high blood pressure and cholesterol.

Acknowledge that each body is a unique creation, wonderfully made, and one-size-fits-all solutions are not the pathway to wellness. You need to discover the weight management strategy that harmonizes with your body's rhythm. Tailoring your approach ensures that it aligns with your metabolic profile, lifestyle, and even your tastes.

Embarking on the journey of weight loss is similar to the transformation of water into wine. It is no instantaneous miracle. Rather, it's a gradual change that develops over time, and patience in this process is vital. As your weight descends, you will notice a gradual but steady improvement in your glucose levels—an affirming sign that your efforts are bearing fruit.

Do not overlook the gravity of mental fortitude in this quest. The mind is a battlefield, and thoughts can either be arrows of doubt or shields of conviction. As you focus on weight management, guarding your heart and mind is imperative because conviction leads to consistency, and consistency paves the way to success.

Another aspect to consider is the interplay between medication and weight. Some diabetes medications might contribute to weight gain, while others may promote weight loss. It's akin to choosing the correct tool for a task; the right medication can make your efforts more effective.

It's critical to view weight management not as a finite conquest with a clear end but as an ongoing voyage. It's about adjusting the sails—diet and activity level—not about waiting for the wind to change. Even upon reaching your target weight, the journey doesn't end there; maintaining that weight requires continued perseverance and adaptation.

Furthermore, the foods you choose to eat play a tremendous role in your weight and blood sugar control. Just as manna from heaven provided nourishment in the wilderness, selecting whole, nutrient-dense foods provides your body with sustenance without excess calories that can lead to weight gain.

Exercise is yet another piece of this intricate puzzle. Physical activity is like the staff that parted the Red Sea—it can create a path toward improved health by increasing insulin sensitivity, aiding weight loss, and boosting your overall well-being.

Reflect on the story of creation and remember that your body is made with intention and purpose. Addressing your weight is not merely a way of bending to societal expectations – it is about respecting the incredible design and capabilities of your own body and taking charge of your health so you may have life, and have it abundantly.

Be gentle with yourself in this process. As seasons change, so might your weight, but let neither define your identity. You are not the number on the scale; you are the perseverance in your spirit, the fortitude in your resolve, and the reflection of the divine image in which you were made.

Finally, invite wisdom into your journey of weight management. Seek knowledge from reputable sources, consult healthcare professionals, and do not rush the process. True wisdom leads to action, and informed action breeds results. As you gain understanding about the impact of weight on diabetes control, let that insight lead you to a healthier, more balanced way of living.

Strategies for Effective Weight Loss As we explore the weight management connection in combatting type 2 diabetes, it is essential to focus on the role weight loss can play in controlling this condition. Often, carrying extra weight strains the body's ability to regulate blood sugar, making diabetes management more challenging. But take heed, for there is wisdom in approaching weight loss with strategies that not only shed pounds but also nourish the body and soul.

In the scriptures of life, patience is often lauded as a virtue, and this certainly holds true when charting a course for effective weight loss. Incremental changes are the stones upon which your path to success is built. Set achievable goals that inspire and motivate you without setting the stage for disappointment. A loss of one to two pounds per week is not just a healthy target; it is a sustainable one, allowing the body to adjust naturally to a new equilibrium.

Consider also the power of dietary wisdom. Just as Daniel chose vegetables and water over the king's delicacies, opting for a diet abundant in vegetables, fruits, lean proteins, and whole grains can lead you towards a healthier weight and improved blood sugar levels. Ensure that your nutritional blueprint includes portion control, for it isn't only what we eat but also how much we consume that can tip the scales.

"Do you not know that your body is a temple of the Holy Spirit?" wrote Paul to the Corinthians. In nurturing this temple, we should engage in regular physical activity that goes beyond our routine tasks. Exercise acts as a catalyst, improving insulin sensitivity, and supporting weight loss efforts. Find activities that resonate with your spirit: walking, swimming, cycling, or perhaps a dance class that elevates both your heart rate and spirits.

Furthermore, embrace consistency. Just as the changing seasons are steadfast, so too should be your approach to eating and exercise. Cultivate a structured mealtime and workout schedule. This repetition breeds habit, and habit forms the backbone of long-lasting change. Do not discount the importance of sleep, for it is the night that knits up the ravell'd sleeve of care. Adequate rest supports metabolic health and helps regulate hormones that affect appetite.

Monitoring your progress is a pillar of weight loss. Every milestone, no matter how small, is like a stone cast upon the waters, creating ripples that reflect your journey. Use a food diary or an app to keep track of your food intake and exercise routine. Periodic reflection will reveal patterns, highlight achievements, and illuminate areas in need of adjustment.

For those moments when temptation beckons and the path seems steep, recall that even "The Lord is my shepherd; I shall not want." Learning to navigate environmental cues and emotional eating involves understanding the triggers that lead to poor food choices and developing strategies to counteract them. Perhaps it will be a matter of seeking solace in prayer, meditation, or conversation rather than in the fleeting satisfaction of comfort foods.

Enlist allies on this journey. Solomon wrote, "Two are better than one, because they have a good return for their labor." A support team consisting of family, friends, healthcare providers, and possibly a dietitian or a personal trainer can provide encouragement and accountability, propelling you forward when your resolve may falter.

Never underestimate the influence of hydration. Water is emblematic of purity and life, and ensuring that you consume ample fluids can help with weight loss and metabolic regulation. Sometimes, what feels like hunger is actually thirst. Before reaching for a snack, drink a glass of water and reassess your body's signals.

Your diet should not be a rigid cage but rather a flexible framework that accommodates interruptions and special occasions. It's not necessary to forsake all treats; balance is key. Permit yourself an occasional indulgence, a feast in a famine for the sake of joy, as long as it does not become the norm. Celebrate your cultural heritage and family traditions with wisdom and moderation.

The renewing of your mind is also critical in this undertaking. Cultivate positive self-talk and set aside self-criticism. Rejoice in your efforts and progress, and remember that each day is a new opportunity to live in accordance with your cherished values and health goals. As the old adage goes, "For as he thinketh in his heart, so is he." Believe in your capacity for change, and it will manifest.

Prepare for setbacks, for they will come. Just as Job faced his trials, so must you face the temporary barriers in your weight loss journey. Do not see them as failures but as learning opportunities. Review what led to the setback, adjust your plan, and have faith that perseverance will bring you closer to your goal.

Finally, weight loss medication may be another stone you can use to strengthen the foundation of your health. In concert with a healthy diet and regular exercise, medication prescribed by a healthcare provider can assist those who have difficulty losing weight through lifestyle changes alone.

Let us not grow weary while doing good, for in due season we shall reap if we do not lose heart. Effective weight loss is not defined solely by the number on the scale, but also by the fortitude of your spirit and the healthfulness of your body. Embrace these strategies with resilience and hope, for they forge the path to not just weight management, but a life more abundant.

As we prepare to delve into tackling weight plateaus in the next section, remember that each step on this journey matters. The road to effective weight loss is one marked by wisdom, patience, and the unwavering belief that you can triumph over adversity and live vibrantly with diabetes.

Dealing with Weight Plateaus When you embark on a journey to better health, especially after a diagnosis of type 2 diabetes, weight management is often an essential chapter. It's a path marked with triumphs and challenges, but perhaps one of the most trying moments is the encounter with a weight plateau. A plateau, often the valley between peaks on your health pilgrimage, can stir a mix of emotions and even self-doubt.

But let's pause and reflect for a moment. The scriptures say, "Consider it pure joy, my brothers and sisters, whenever you face trials of many kinds" (James 1:2). Now, while weight plateaus aren't necessarily a trial of faith, they're an opportunity for growth. They teach us to persevere and find strength in places we didn't know existed. It's in these periods of stillness that the roots of our resolve deepen, providing the strength to push through to the other side.

Understanding that weight plateaus are a normal and temporary part of the weight loss process is crucial. They're a sign that your body is adjusting and finding a new equilibrium. It's a complex system that seeks balance, and as you lose weight, your metabolism begins to adapt. This adaptation is a testament to the incredible design of our bodies but also a call to refine our strategies.

Let's talk about dealing with these plateaus constructively. First, recall the goal is not just to lose weight, but to nurture a body that's strong, resilient, and better equipped to manage diabetes. This isn't about rapid transformations, but lasting change. Approach each day with fresh vigor, understanding that "patience must finish its work so that you may be mature and complete, not lacking anything" (James 1:4).

To break through a plateau, consider adjusting your nutritional blueprint. It might be time to reassess your caloric intake and ensure it aligns with your current weight and activity level. Sometimes, a small decrease in calories or a slight alteration in your macros can restart the weight loss process. It's also valuable to revisit your meal plan and incorporate new diabetes-friendly recipes that could reignite your metabolism's fire.

Exercise, too, plays a pivotal role in surmounting the weight plateau. If your routine has become monotonous, inject new life into it. Vary your exercises, increase the intensity, or add another day of workouts into your week. Muscle bears the honor of torching calories more efficiently than fat, so consider incorporating strength training to build lean muscle mass.

It's also beneficial to record your journey meticulously. Maintain food diaries and exercise logs; they can reveal patterns or habits you might overlook. Sometimes, the devil is in the details—seemingly innocent calorie creep or a reduction in physical activity can silently sabotage weight loss efforts.

One often overlooked aspect is sleep and stress management. Chronic stress and sleep deprivation can lead to hormonal imbalances which may hinder weight loss. The hormonal interplay within our bodies is intricate, and when cortisol levels rise due to stress, this can trigger an increase in appetite and fat storage, particularly around the midsection.

Mindfulness in eating and living is a potent tool. Take the time to savor your meals, to eat slowly with gratitude, recognizing each bite as nourishment. Mindfulness helps you listen to your body's signals of hunger and fullness, thereby reducing the likelihood of emotional eating which can contribute to plateaus.

Don't forget to hydrate. Water plays an invaluable role in metabolism and hunger regulation. Sometimes, thirst masks itself as hunger, leading to unnecessary snacking. Drinking a sufficient amount of water keeps your body's systems flowing smoothly and aids in breaking down fat for energy.

As you maneuver through this plateau, remember that the measure of success isn't just the falling numbers on a scale, but also the rise in your ability to manage diabetes more effectively. Celebrate non-scale victories like better blood sugar readings, enhanced fitness levels, or even the simple joy of walking up stairs without shortness of breath. These milestones are tangible evidence of your commitment to health.

If months pass and the plateau remains steadfast, consult with your healthcare team. They can help identify any underlying issues and may adjust your medication or recommend other interventions.

Yet, the greatest tool at your disposal is the perseverance of the human spirit. Embody the wisdom that "perseverance must finish its work so that you may be mature and complete, not lacking anything" (James 1:4). Approach each day as a new opportunity to reinforce your commitment to health, and regard each obstacle as a lesson to learn and grow from.

Be encouraged that plateaus are temporary. With patience, persistence, and a willingness to adapt your approach, you'll find yourself breaking through to new heights. Your journey is unique and sacred, a testament to the strength within you to overcome. As you press on, remember that each step, even those that seem stationary, is moving you forward towards a healthier, more vibrant life.

In summary, as you navigate weight plateaus, do so with the understanding that they are not signs of failure, but rather intricate parts of a larger story—one of growth, adaptation, and ultimate triumph. In the stillness of these plateaus, dig deep to find the strength and wisdom to ascend again, and rejoice in the knowledge that every challenge surmounted enriches your journey and brings you one step closer to living in harmony with diabetes.

Chapter 7:
Living with Diabetes: Day-to-Day Strategies

In navigating the landscape of life with diabetes, each dawn offers new mercies and challenges alike. The daily bread of managing this condition requires consistent, practical strategies that foster wellbeing amidst the ebb and flow of glucose levels. Sustaining harmony between vigilance and grace, one develops an intimate dance with the nuances of their body's needs. Unseen victories are won through regular patterns of mindfulness during mundane moments, like choosing water over sugary drinks or taking the stairs with praise for the strength to ascend. Whether journeying cross-country or confronting a common cold, those who walk with diabetes tread with an awareness that their path, though sprinkled with trials, is lit with hope and the empowerment that comes from a day seized with intention. Embodying the wisdom of ancient text, one learns to number their days with insight, acknowledging the preciousness of life's moments, and fostering the resilience to meet each day's demands with a steadfast heart.

Managing Highs and Lows As we navigate the everyday intricacies of living with diabetes, we are constantly reminded that life is a balancing act, an endeavor of maintaining equilibrium amidst a myriad of changes. For those with type 2 diabetes, managing the fluctuations in blood glucose levels becomes a central pillar of daily self-care. In this section, we shall explore practical strategies and philosophies that embolden us to steer through these highs and lows with grace and wisdom.

The journey through diabetes is not one of smooth sailing; there will be tempests and calm seas alike. It's vital to remember that both hyperglycemia (high blood glucose) and hypoglycemia (low blood glucose) come with signs that beckon our attention. Recognizing these signals early can be the difference between tranquility and turmoil. As Proverbs 4:6-7 teaches us, "Do not forsake wisdom, and she will protect you; love her, and she will watch over you. The beginning of wisdom is this: Get wisdom. Though it cost all you have, get understanding." In this context, wisdom lies in attuning oneself to the body's cues and responding with both knowledge and discernment.

Hyperglycemia can manifest through symptoms such as excessive thirst, frequent urination, fatigue, and blurred vision. If left unmanaged, it can lead to severe complications. Conversely, hypoglycemia may present as dizziness, sweating, confusion, or shakiness. It's imperative to know that every individual with diabetes may experience a unique blend of these symptoms, and thus one's vigilance in self-monitoring becomes paramount.

To manage highs, dietary discipline plays a significant role. Consuming balanced meals with appropriate portions of carbohydrates, fiber, protein, and healthy fats can help stabilize blood glucose levels. Moreover, being mindful of the glycemic index of foods can provide additional guidance in meal planning. "Man shall not live by bread alone, but by every word that comes from the mouth of God" (Matthew 4:4), reminds us that nourishment extends beyond the physical; it encompasses the wisdom of informed dietary choices.

Amidst high blood sugars, it's crucial not to neglect one's medication regime. Medications are a divine provision akin to manna from heaven, provided to assist in the management of our condition.

Consistent medication, in harmony with lifestyle adjustments, forms the cornerstone of effective diabetes control.

When grappling with low blood sugars, one must act swiftly to restore balance. The 'rule of 15'—consuming 15 grams of fast-acting carbohydrates and checking blood sugar after 15 minutes—is a practical approach supported by health professionals. It encapsulates the sage advice to "let all things be done decently and in order" (1 Corinthians 14:40), further highlighting the importance of methodical responses to such instances.

Equally important is the practice of regular blood glucose monitoring. This discipline serves as a mirror, reflecting the real-time status of our condition, and is vital for making informed decisions about diet, exercise, and medication. Embrace this task with the kind of diligence Proverbs 21:5 praises: "The plans of the diligent lead surely to abundance, but everyone who is hasty comes only to poverty."

Remember, fluctuations in blood sugar levels are not failures but rather moments to learn and apply newfound knowledge. Self-compassion should be your companion on this journey, for it is written, "Therefore, as God's chosen people, holy and dearly loved, clothe yourselves with compassion, kindness, humility, gentleness, and patience" (Colossians 3:12). In practicing self-forgiveness and understanding, we open the door for continuous improvement.

Managing diabetes also means being aware of how exercise affects blood glucose levels. Physical activity typically lowers blood sugar, so it's important to consume a small carbohydrate-based snack beforehand if levels are on the lower end, or to adjust medication as advised by your healthcare provider. Yet, exercise is not only good for the body but the spirit as well. The scripture reminds us to "train yourself for godliness" (1 Timothy 4:7), and in this training, our physical bodies are included as temples.

Stress, surprisingly, can cause both spikes and drops in glucose levels. Learning stress-reduction techniques such as deep breathing, meditation, or yoga can be highly beneficial. Philippians 4:6-7 encourages us in saying, "Do not be anxious about anything, but in every situation, by prayer and petition, with thanksgiving, present your requests to God." Taking this to heart within the context of diabetes management, one finds peace not only in spiritual realms but in physical manifestation through stabilized glucose readings.

Nighttime management is equally worth noting. Ensuring a balanced meal in the evening and considering a bedtime snack with proteins may prevent overnight blood sugar lows. Just as the Psalmist found solace in God's presence at night, saying, "In peace I will lie down and sleep, for you alone, LORD, make me dwell in safety" (Psalm 4:8), you too can rest more securely knowing you have prepared your body for a steady night.

Moreover, it is advisable to educate close family members or friends on how to recognize and react to severe hypoglycemia, should you be unable to do so yourself. Equip your loved ones with the knowledge to be your guardian angels, illustratively extending the biblical principle of "bearing one another's burdens" (Galatians 6:2) into the realm of practical care and support.

Lastly, maintaining meticulous records of your blood glucose levels, medications, meals, and activities can serve as a guide to understanding the patterns of your diabetes management over time. This is akin to keeping a faithful account of one's journey of faith, marking the ebb and flow, gaining insight and foresight that only comes from reflection and review.

As we come to a close on this topic, it's essential to integrate these principles and practices with steadfastness and hope. Remember that the highs and lows are but waves on the vast ocean of life. Just as Jesus calmed the storm, saying, "Peace! Be still!" (Mark 4:39), so too can you find serenity amidst the fluctuations of diabetes by managing wisely and living fully.

In summary, managing the highs and lows of type 2 diabetes is a multifaceted undertaking that requires awareness, education, and proactive approaches. Embrace the journey not with trepidation but with an eye towards growth and strength. As you implement these strategies, may you forge ahead with resilience, upheld by the knowledge that steadiness awaits across the undulating waves of this condition.

Traveling with Diabetes As we continue our exploration of thriving with type 2 diabetes, we venture into a realm full of excitement and potential anxiety: travel. The freedom to traverse borders and discover new horizons is not diminished by your diagnosis. Yet, it calls for an extra layer of preparation and mindfulness to ensure your journey is not just safe, but also enjoyable.

Embarking on travel requires thoughtful consideration and planning for everyone, but for those with diabetes, it carries a deeper significance. Each step of the journey, much like the path of life, presents opportunities to trust in your preparation and adaptability. As Proverbs 16:9 guides us, "The heart of man plans his way, but the Lord establishes his steps." This principle rings true as you prepare for travel; plan diligently, yet hold the awareness that flexibility and trust in oneself are key.

Prior to departure, consult with your healthcare provider to ensure your diabetes management plan is suited for the demands of travel. This may encompass temporary adjustments to your medication regimen in light of time zone changes or activity levels. Like the children of Israel who trusted in God's pillar of cloud and fire, let your healthcare provider's advice be your guide to navigate this new terrain.

Packing for travel becomes an exercise in foresight. You'll need to pack not just enough medication and supplies for the duration of your trip, but also a contingency surplus. Consider the story of the five wise virgins in Matthew 25, who brought extra oil for their lamps, ensuring they were prepared for any eventuality. In the same vein, bring extra supplies to light your way, should your journey stretch beyond anticipated.

Whether crossing vast oceans or winding through country roads, keep your medications and supplies close at hand. In the event of lost luggage, a carry-on with your essentials is your David's sling against a Goliath-sized headache. Carry a letter from your doctor explaining your condition and treatment as your shield of legitimacy if questioned by authorities.

When navigating the airport or long stretches on the road, regular blood glucose monitoring remains crucial. Ponder the wisdom of Ecclesiastes 3:1, "For everything there is a season, and a time for every matter under heaven." Just as there is a time to sow and a time to reap, there is a time to check and a time to act, ensuring your blood sugar stays within the safe harbors of control.

Nutrition while traveling can appear like a serpentine path, temptingly filled with the unknown. Just as Daniel refused the king's rich food, standing true to his dietary needs, remain steadfast in seeking out options in line with your nutritional blueprint.

As air travel can lead to periods of prolonged inactivity, be like Paul, who spoke of 'running the race' in 1 Corinthians 9:24. Find ways to keep your physical activity consistent, even if that means walking the airport terminal or stretching at rest stops. Your body will reward you with better blood sugar management, and your spirit with an invigorated sense of well-being.

Time zone transitions can disrupt your usual medication schedule. Just as the wise men watched the stars for signs, watch the clock for cues to adjust your routine. Staying in tune with your body's signals will help you recalibrate as you move across meridians.

Dining out is an integral part of travel and exploration. Rather than a mountain of dietary temptation, see it as a valley of decision. Examine menus as you would a map, selecting routes that align with your health goals. Asking for nutritional information may seem daunting, but it is a small act of courage with a great reward.

In foreign lands, the language barrier can pose a challenge like the Tower of Babel. Consider using technology such as translation apps, or carrying a card that explains your diabetes in the local language. This prepares you to communicate crucial information, breakdown walls of confusion, and receive the assistance you may need.

Sometimes travel brings unforeseen hardships, akin to Paul's shipwreck on Malta. Should you face such challenges, seek out local pharmacies or hospitals. Your preparation and persistence, as displayed by Paul, will guide you to safety and support in even the most turbulent of circumstances.

As fatigue may set in, remember Elijah's exhaustion under the broom tree. Sometimes, you may need to rest and refuel your body and spirit with proper nourishment and sleep. Rest is not a sign of weakness but an acknowledgment of one's humanity and need for renewal, ensuring you can savor each moment of your journey.

Throughout your travels, keep close contact with your support team back home. Modern technology allows you the privilege of seeking guidance through video calls or messaging, much like the early church stayed connected through epistles. This network of support will buoy your spirit and provide assistance when needed.

I travel frequently and one of the biggest challenges is keeping up with my regiment while on the road. I actually prefer to drive when I travel and have found a number of products that make my travels a bit more convenient. If you'd like to take a look at some of these products, they will be listed with links on my corporate website www.MyMaverickWorld.com.

Finally, reflect on your travel experiences as a microcosm of your larger journey with diabetes. Each city visited, every cuisine sampled, and all the challenges faced are brushstrokes in the masterpiece that is your life. Enriched by these experiences, you return home not just with souvenirs but with a deeper understanding of your own strength and capability in managing diabetes, no matter where life takes you.

Coping with Sick Days Living with diabetes involves navigating through the ebbs and flows of daily life with a meticulous mindset, especially when sick days emerge. Illness can be a tumultuous period for anyone, but when you're managing type 2 diabetes, the stakes are considerably higher. Viral infections, the common cold, or even digestive issues can send your blood sugar levels on an unpredictable journey.

It is in these times of physical ailment that the strength of human spirit, intertwined with wisdom, is most crucial. Biblical principles encourage perseverance through adversity, and in addressing health, they often advocate for a mindset of stewardship over one's body. As you face the trials of sickness, consider your body a temple, and act with intention to restore it to health.

The first step to being prepared for sick days starts well before any symptoms appear. Establishing a routine for blood glucose monitoring is paramount. When illness strikes, your body reacts by releasing stress hormones to fight the infection, often leading to rising blood sugar levels, despite eating less or having an altered appetite.

Maintaining hydration is crucial during these trying times. The human body, much like the earth, is composed predominantly of water, and its flowing nature is essential for life. Adequate fluid intake helps to thin mucus, supports kidney function, and aids in preventing dehydration—a risk that can be compounded by high blood sugar.

Reflect on the guidance of Philippians 4:6-7, "Do not be anxious about anything..." and apply this to your approach to managing diabetes on sick days. Worrying can increase stress levels, thereby affecting blood glucose. Instead, be prepared to pivot your management strategies, and maintain an open line of communication with your healthcare provider.

Healthy eating can become challenging when you're not feeling your best, yet it's vital to continue nourishing your body. Small, manageable meals or snacks that are consistent with your dietary plan are important. Think of the biblical analogy of daily bread—seek sustenance that gives strength and aligns with the body's need for balance.

There's also the matter of medication. When your daily routine is thrown off by sickness, so too might be the timing and effect of your medications. Keep in close contact with your healthcare team to adjust dosages if necessary—this may include both diabetes medications and any over-the-counter remedies for your sickness symptoms.

Recording your symptoms and blood glucose levels becomes even more essential when you're sick. This log provides a narrative, a map that reveals the impact of illness on your body's balance. In the Scriptural sense, it is like maintaining a written testament of a challenging journey, providing insights that can guide future actions.

During this period of vulnerability, do not shy away from asking for help. Whether it's for assistance in running errands, preparing food, or just having someone to check in on you, seek out your support network. In this, reflect on the parable of the Good Samaritan—embodying the comfort and compassion one should find in community.

It's important to recognize when an illness is more than just a passing discomfort and when professional medical attention is necessary. High fever, persistent vomiting, or signs of dehydration are all pits in the road that may require additional aid to navigate.

Rest is another pivotal element in combating sickness and managing diabetes. It allows the body to repair and restore itself—a physical embodiment of seeking peace and surrendering one's anxieties and ailments to a higher power. Rest without guilt, as it is necessary for healing.

If you're on insulin, be prepared to possibly adjust your insulin regimen under the guidance of your healthcare professional. Remember, insulin can sometimes be required more during illness, even if you are eating less than usual.

On the flip side, avoid the trap of self-isolation during sick days. Keeping your emotional and spiritual health aligned with your physical health is essential. Ecclesiastes 4:9-10 speaks to the power of companionship and the importance of having someone to help when one falls—your emotional wellbeing is deeply interconnected with your physical recovery.

Lastly, reflect upon what has worked and what hasn't after you have recovered. A strategic review of your coping mechanisms during sick days gravitates toward a philosophy of continuous improvement. Like refining gold through fire, each sickness can teach you more about managing your diabetes with grace and wisdom.

Embrace each sick day as an opportunity for growth and learning. Remind yourself that your journey with diabetes is one of courage and resilience, walking a path paved with challenges, but also triumphs.

Remember that with each step, you're not alone. You are equipped, supported, and capable. May the peace that surpasses all understanding guard your hearts and your bodies, as you journey on to vibrant health and well-being.

Chapter 8:
Beyond the Physical: Mental Health and Coping

As we've journeyed thus far, we've meticulously carved a path through the multi-faceted world of living with type 2 diabetes, addressing the tangible aspects of nutrition, exercise, and day-to-day management. Now, we venture into the realm where the silent battles wage—the mind. The challenge of diabetes isn't just the physical rigor; it's equally a test of emotional and psychological fortitude. Understanding that the body and the spirit are inextricably linked is a revelation that carries the power to transform. One of the reasons that I started thinking about actually writing this book was when a friend that I had known for more than 35 years, passed away from diabetes. The emotional and mental challenges can be really tough and this was a wakeup call for me on the emotional effects of diabetes. In this chapter, we will confront the specter of diabetes burnout with wisdom, intercept cycles of anxiety and emotional eating with grace, and fortify our resilience as we seek and extend support. It's here, in recognizing mental health as a pivotal component of diabetes management, where we learn not just to cope, but to thrive in harmony with our conditions. Let us hold fast the conviction that wellness transcends the physical shell, and that in nurturing our inner strength, we kindle a flame that the fiercest of storms can't extinguish.

Dealing with Diabetes Burnout As you navigate life with type 2 diabetes, it is not uncommon to encounter periods of exhaustion and frustration - times when the relentless daily management feels overwhelming. You've monitored your blood sugar, tailored your diet, kept up with exercise, and stayed vigilant with your medication, and yet, the weight of responsibility persists, growing heavy. This, my friends, is diabetes burnout, a state where even the most resilient spirits find themselves flagging. But take heart; for every challenge we face, there lies a scripture of hope, a philosophical insight, or an inspirational tale to uplift us.

Consider the analogy of the potter and the clay. As people with diabetes, we are both the potter and the clay, continually shaping and being shaped by our experiences with this chronic condition. Burnout can feel like the clay has gone dry, hard to mold, and resistant to change. Let us then find the living waters that rejuvenate the spirit – through self-care, compassion, and renewed purpose.

The biblical imperative to 'not grow weary in doing good' reflects upon the long-term nature of managing diabetes. Even when your strength wanes, know that it is in perseverance that character is built and hope is found. Reflecting upon the stoic wisdom, remind yourself that it is not the situation itself but our reaction to it that defines our path. Take a breath, pause, and acknowledge your efforts, for they are not in vain.

One practical step in overcoming burnout is to simplify your diabetes management routine. Examine the processes you have set in place; are there steps you can streamline? Perhaps technology can assist with monitoring, or maybe there are meal prep tricks that save time without compromising on nutrition. In simplification, you may find a path that is less burdensome and more sustainable.

Next, bring mindfulness into your daily regimen. Mindfulness is the art of being present and fully engaging with the task at hand. When checking blood sugar levels or preparing a meal, avoid going through the motions mindlessly. Be present in that moment, focusing on your well-being and the empowering choice you are making towards a healthier you.

Seek to kindle joy in the small victories. Each day you successfully manage your diabetes is a testament to your strength. Embrace a philosophy of celebrating the little things, whether it be a favorable blood glucose reading, a brisk walk in the open air, or mastering a new diabetes-friendly recipe. Let gratitude be the fuel that reignites your passion for self-care.

The therapeutic act of creating something tangible cannot be overstated. Engage in activities unconnected to diabetes that bring you satisfaction, whether it be gardening, painting, or crafting. These acts not only provide a respite but remind you that you are multifaceted, more than your diagnosis.

Reconnect with your community. Surrounding yourself with people who understand your journey can be incredibly uplifting. Attend local support groups or find online forums where you can share your struggles and your triumphs. There is solace in shared experience and strength in unity.

Trust that it is okay to ask for help. This is not an admission of defeat; rather, it is an affirmation that you value your well-being. Reach out to healthcare professionals or counselors who specialize in chronic illness management. Their guidance can offer a fresh perspective and renew your energy to continue your fight against diabetes.

Reflection, too, holds the power to transform weariness into wisdom. Reflect upon your journey with diabetes thus far. Acknowledge not only the hardships but also how far you've come. You've braved storms and relished in calm seas. This reflection can serve as an internal compass, guiding you through current and future challenges.

Another tactic in your arsenal against burnout is to imbue your routine with flexibility. Rigidity can become stifling. Allow yourself the grace to make adjustments when needed, whether it be in your diet, exercise, or medication. This isn't a sign of weakness but an example of adaptive strength.

Educate yourself, but do so judiciously. An influx of information can be as overwhelming as ignorance. Balance is key; learn about your condition and its management in ways that empower rather than overload you. A measured approach to education can be a source of comfort and control.

Occasionally, taking a break is necessary – not from caring for your diabetes, but from the emotional weight of it. Give yourself permission to set aside the stresses for a moment. During this time of rest, lean into your faith or your personal philosophy for solace, drawing on these resolute pillars for the peace that surpasses all understanding.

And finally, envision a future unfettered by current frustrations. Hope is an intrinsic human trait, deep-seated and tenacious. Foster this hope by setting small, achievable goals that lead to larger aspirations. It's in the quiet unfolding of each day that our lives are woven into a tapestry of triumphs and trials, each thread significant and telling a story of resilience.

Remember, managing diabetes is a lifelong journey, and it's natural to encounter periods where the road feels steep and the burden heavy. Yet within you lies an invincible summer, a vibrant spirit ready to rise anew. As you face diabetes burnout, embrace these strategies, lean on your faith and philosophy, and, with renewed vigor, continue the noble endeavor of nurturing your well-being.

Anxiety, Depression, and Emotional Eating may not be the first concerns that come to mind following a type 2 diabetes diagnosis. Yet, as you travel this journey, it's evident that the tidal waves of emotional upheaval can profoundly impact dietary choices and well-being. Understanding the intricate relationship between your mental health and eating habits is crucial for sustaining a life filled with hope and vitality in the face of diabetes.

When the word 'anxiety' slips into the conversation, it might conjure up images of restless nights and incessant worry. For many living with diabetes, anxiety can stem from the constant monitoring of blood sugar levels, fear of complications, or even the pressure of maintaining strict dietary regimens. Anxiety's grip can be paralyzing, making it harder to stay committed to health-promoting behaviors.

Depression, a close companion to anxiety, often walks hand-in-hand with chronic illnesses like diabetes. The overwhelming sensation that engulfs you, casting shadows on joy and draining the color from life's tapestry, is more than a mere feeling of sadness—it's a serious health condition that requires attention and care.

Together, anxiety and depression can pave the way for emotional eating—a coping strategy where food becomes the salve for soothing emotional wounds. It's the reach for sweet comfort or the crunch of frustration, where the act of eating serves to fill emotional voids rather than physical hunger. Emotional eating can disrupt the delicate balance of a diabetes-friendly diet and complicate blood sugar control.

Understanding that the body, mind, and spirit are woven into a tapestry of interconnected strands can guide you through these emotional challenges. Remember, you are not alone on this pilgrimage. The valleys of despair can give way to peaks of courage and strength, as told within the Psalms, offering a reminder that hope and support are ever-present.

Food, while nourishing, can become a double-edged sword. The act of eating should be a reflection of self-care, not self-sabotage. It's important to pause and reflect on whether hunger is the true cause of your cravings or if deeper emotional currents are at play. Strategies such as mindful eating, where you engage all senses and savor each bite, can be an act of worship, a moment to express gratitude for the sustenance provided by our Creator.

To confront anxiety and depression, an arsenal of tools can be wielded. Prayer and meditation can anchor the soul, offering peace amidst the storm. The regular practice of these spiritual disciplines can calm the heart and center the mind, providing clarity and focus to manage diabetes effectively.

Regular physical activity is another potent antidote to the poison of anxiety and depression. As you engage in exercise, the body releases endorphins—chemicals that act as natural painkillers and mood elevators. Exercise becomes not only a means to improve physical health but also a rhythmic dance of perseverance that uplifts the spirit.

Cultivating a support network is of paramount importance. Speaking with friends, joining a support group, or consulting with a mental health professional can provide a lifeline during turbulent times. It's in these relationships that burdens are shared, and the yoke of diabetes can be lightened, as the Scripture encourages us to bear one another's burdens.

Partaking in the bread of understanding, finding joy in nourishment rather than solace in indulgence, rekindles the spirit's flame. When emotional eating beckons, seek wholesome alternatives that satisfy the body without derailing your diabetes management. Lean on the wisdom of Proverbs, which teaches us that prudence is a fountain of life, enabling you to make enlightened choices for your well-being.

Should you stumble, practice forgiveness—extend to yourself the same grace you would to others. Missteps are not failures but opportunities for growth and learning. As you find strength in forgiveness, you build resilience, a fortress against the storms of anxiety and depression.

Documentation, such as maintaining a food diary as discussed in Appendix B, can aid in identifying patterns of emotional eating. This act of reflection isn't about casting judgment but observing with kindness and gaining insight into how emotions influence eating behaviors.

It's through these trials that character is refined. As gold is tested in fire, so too are you, emerging purer and stronger. Confronting the challenges of anxiety, depression, and emotional eating not only builds your endurance but also deepens your compassion for others traveling this path.

In the harmonious balance of body, mind, and spirit, there is healing. A diabetes diagnosis may seem a formidable foe, but it also presents an opportunity to grow in ways never imagined. Embrace this path with courage, knowing the strength you glean from this battle can inspire and illuminate the way for others.

As you draw this section to a close, look inward and be encouraged. Your journey with diabetes is more than managing a physical condition—it's a spiritual quest that, with care and compassion, can transform your life. In the light of understanding and with a heart full of faith, stride forward. You are more than your diagnosis; you are a testimony of endurance, a beacon of hope, a testament to the resilience of the human spirit.

Building Resilience and Seeking Support As individuals journey through life with Type 2 diabetes, an essential component of managing the condition is building resilience and actively seeking support. Cultivating a resilient spirit enables one to weather the inevitable storms and adapt to the changing tides that accompany this diagnosis. But what does building resilience truly entail, and how can it be fortified alongside a network of support?

Resilience is often likened to the steadfastness of a tree in a tempest - bending, but never breaking. To cultivate such endurance in your life, begin by focusing on the foundational roots: mindset, education, and the acceptance of change. A mindset anchored in hope and optimism fortifies you against despair, as the Apostle Paul encourages, "Be joyful in hope, patient in affliction, faithful in prayer" (Romans 12:12). Embrace education as your shield; understanding your condition empowers you to make informed decisions. Acceptance allows you to adapt to new circumstances with grace rather than resistance.

Finding strength within yourself is paramount, but so is seeking the strength that lies in togetherness. Building your support team as outlined in earlier chapters is the first step. Dive deeper by joining diabetes support groups, whether local or online. In these gatherings, you'll find others walking similar paths, ready to share their insights, struggles, and victories. Here, the biblical principle "As iron sharpens iron, so one person sharpens another" (Proverbs 27:17) comes to life, with peers uplifting and refining one another through shared experiences.

Moreover, don't overlook the value of professional support. Therapists, counselors, and diabetes educators provide a scaffolding of guidance, helping to navigate the emotional and practical complexities of living with diabetes. They are akin to the reinforcements that steady a ship during a storm, offering not just solace but strategies to maintain your course.

Practicing self-care is a further expression of resilience. Prioritize activities that nourish your soul, such as meditation, prayer, or participating in a beloved hobby. These moments of rejuvenation are crucial, allowing you to "renew your strength... [to] soar on wings like eagles" (Isaiah 40:31). Remember, the care you afford yourself is not a luxury, but a necessity.

One must also learn the art of self-advocacy in the healthcare system. This means being assertive about your needs, asking probing questions, and demanding the best care possible. Like David facing Goliath, with knowledge as your sling and determination as your stone, you can conquer what may seem insurmountable.

Challenges with diabetes are interoperable, with physical, emotional, and spiritual dimensions. When blood sugars fluctuate, for example, it may not only be a physical alert but an emotional signal, too. It's a call to assess not just your diet but also your stress levels and emotional well-being. Resilience involves this holistic approach, recognizing the interconnectedness of your experiences.

Resilient individuals also acknowledge their triumphs. Keeping a journal of your successes, no matter how small, builds a reservoir of positive reflections for harder days. Use these as reminders of your perseverance, like stones of remembrance used by the Israelites after crossing into the Promised Land (Joshua 4:6-7), markers of victory on your journey with diabetes.

Never underestimate the strength that can be drawn from setting goals. Whether they're related to blood sugar levels, exercise, or nutritional achievements, goals give you a roadmap for your journey. As Jesus said with the parable of the talents (Matthew 25:14-30), it is by using well what we have that we are entrusted with more. Regarding your health, the principle stands: steward your body faithfully by setting and pursuing attainable goals.

The resilience you build is not a static fortress, but a dynamic ecosystem. It evolves as you learn more about your diabetes, as you encounter life's changes, and as you deepen your spiritual roots. Like the new wineskins that Jesus spoke of (Luke 5:37-38), you must be flexible and ready to contain the new wine—new experiences, knowledge, and wisdom—that life pours into you.

When moments of discouragement inevitably come, reach out to your support system. Remember Moses, whose arms were held up by Aaron and Hur during battle (Exodus 17:12), illustrating how vital the support of others is to our victories. Your healthcare team, family, friends, and support groups can all play the part of Aaron and Hur, lifting you up when you need it most.

Furthermore, practicing gratitude can enhance resilience. Acknowledge and give thanks for the progress you've made, the people who've supported you, and even the lessons learned through difficulty. Gratitude shifts your perspective, allowing you to see God's grace in your journey and fostering a heart of contentment and strength.

Lastly, remember that your experience living with diabetes can become a source of support and inspiration to others. As you build resilience and grow in your capacity to manage your health, you become a beacon of hope to those starting on their path, or struggling along the way. "Encourage one another and build each other up," (1 Thessalonians 5:11) is not just an instruction but a call to action, using your journey to uplift others.

As this chapter comes to a close, reflect on the ways you've begun to build resilience and the support networks you've established. Take heart that, like a well-tended garden, they will grow and flourish, offering you nourishment and shelter on your journey with diabetes.

Having equipped yourself with strategies to build resilience and seek support, let's prepare to explore the next critical chapter - recognizing complications and learning about vital prevention tactics. This knowledge will serve as your compass, directing you towards continued health, and empowering you to thrive in the face of adversity.

Chapter 9:
Complications and Prevention

In the aftermath of deciphering the complexities of type 2 diabetes, one stands before the twin pillars of vigilance: recognizing potential complications and adamantly pursuing their prevention. As you have armed yourself with nutritional knowledge and emboldened your spirit with exercise, it's imperative to cast a discerning eye on the path ahead. Manifestations of tribulation may arise silently, like shadows at dusk—neuropathy, retinopathy, and cardiovascular machinations threaten the unwary. Yet, these are not inevitable fates inscribed in stone. By intertwining routine check-ups and preventative tests into the tapestry of your life, you construct a fortress against unforeseen ailments. With due attention given to the sanctity of foot and eye care, you are not merely avoiding disaster; you are shepherding your body towards a future where health does not flicker like a candle in the wind, but rather shines steadily like a beacon of hope. Embrace this chapter as your guardian, a lighthouse guiding the vessels of your self-care decisions through misty seas, steering clear of the rocky shallows and navigating towards the tranquility of long-term wellness.

Recognizing and Preventing Long-Term Complications is a pivotal endeavor in the life of an individual with type 2 diabetes. As we journey together through the challenges and revelations of managing diabetes, it becomes clear that diligence and knowledge are our most trusted companions. This chapter seeks to illuminate the path toward understanding and avoiding the prolonged adversities that diabetes can bring.

Long-term complications of diabetes stem from elevated blood sugar levels that persist over an extended period. These can manifest in various forms, impacting numerous systems within the body. Vascular issues may lead to cardiovascular diseases, while nerve damage—also known as diabetic neuropathy—can result in loss of sensation, particularly in the extremities. Over time, the kidneys may be burdened, and the eyes can suffer damage, among other potential issues.

To triumph over these challenges, recognizing the signs is foundational. Subtle changes in one's physical condition, such as tingling sensations in the hands and feet, or fluctuations in vision, should raise your awareness. It is in these details that early indicators of complications may whisper a warning, urging prompt action and intervention.

Prevention, often a tapestry of small yet powerful daily choices, is central to the philosophy of diabetes care. Controlling blood sugar levels within the guidelines provided by healthcare professionals is akin to steering your vessel away from dangerous waters. Dietary prudence, consistent exercise, and medication adherence form a trinity of managing practices that can keep dire long-term complications at bay.

Moreover, regular monitoring of blood glucose and adhering to recommended check-ups provide opportunities for early detection and intervention. These check-ups are not mere appointments but are essential milestones on one's journey to a full and healthful life. They are the watchtowers that alert an individual to oncoming threats before they become visible on the horizon.

The Bible tells us that our bodies are temples, and in the context of diabetes, this truth closely aligns with the practice of routine monitoring and care. Being respecters and stewards of our own temples by doing what is necessary to keep them intact reflects the wisdom of stewardship.

One of the philosophical principles in the fight against diabetes complications is the concept of interconnectedness. Our body's systems are interwoven, and as such, taking comprehensive care of one's cardiovascular health also positively influences other potential complications. For instance, maintaining healthy blood pressure and cholesterol levels can substantially mitigate risk factors.

Staying informed about diabetes and its treatments plays a vital role. Education empowers; it enables one to make choices that align with longevity and vitality. Education is not merely a phase; it is an ongoing practice that evolves as advancements in treatment and understanding of the disease progress.

Additionally, mindfulness of one's mental health creates a bedrock for preventing complications. Stress and anxiety can have tangible effects on glucose levels; thus, a serene spirit and stable mind are not just desirable—they're necessary for optimal physical health.

One must not underestimate the power of community and relationships in bolstering one's resolve to manage diabetes vigilantly. Having allies in the form of healthcare providers, family, and friends to encourage and support, mirrors the biblical ethos of seeking fellowship and unity in the face of adversity.

Motivational dialogues with healthcare professionals are not merely conversations; they are the strategic planning sessions that can help you to chart a course for health success. Individualized care plans, created in partnership with medical teams, ensure that your unique needs are met while navigating the complexities of diabetes.

Adopting healthy lifestyle changes despite the temptations of convenience can be a challenge, yet the satisfaction of knowing you are safeguarding your well-being is an intrinsic reward. This practice speaks to the motivational adage that discipline is choosing between what you want now and what you want most.

It's equally crucial to acknowledge that while prevention is the goal, perfection is not the standard. The journey will have its stumbles, yet the steadfast commitment to rebound and readjust is what defines long-term success. Each day presents a new opportunity to renew this commitment, to continue the journey with wisdom and courage.

In moments of difficulty or discouragement, it is imperative to draw strength from inspirational sources, whether they are spiritual passages, personal mantras, or the support of loved ones. The culmination of these efforts is a life lived not in fear of complications, but with the celebration of the victories gained each day over diabetes.

In closing, let us reflect on the truth that preventing long-term complications necessitates a blend of practical steps and an empowered mindset. As you turn the pages of your life, let each chapter be written with intentionality, informed choices, and a commitment to stewardship over your health. Doing so will not only extend your years but enrich the quality of each day you are granted.

Regular Check-Ups and Tests to Maintain Health are the linchpins that hold your diabetes management plan firmly in place. These periodic evaluations are not just appointments or entries in a calendar; they are milestones on the continuum of care that chart the course of your well-being.

As we journey together in this chapter, consider the scriptural wisdom of being 'watchful'. To manage Type 2 diabetes well, one must be vigilant and proactive with health. Regular check-ups are vital, like the watchmen on the walls, for they provide early warning signs of potential complications.

Your doctor will recommend routine blood tests to keep a close eye on your blood glucose levels. This includes the all-important hemoglobin A1C test which gives a picture of your average blood sugar control over the past two to three months. It is a beacon, guiding the way to understanding how well your management plan is working.

Maintaining a healthy balance of cholesterol levels and blood pressure is also crucial. These tests, often done alongside your A1C, are not mere formalities but signposts that indicate the health of your cardiovascular system, which diabetes can affect over time.

Kidney function tests are another critical component of your regular check-up routine. Diabetes can take a toll on these vital organs, and tests such as the urine albumin test measure the amount of protein in your urine, an indicator of kidney health.

Liver function tests should not be overlooked as well. The liver plays a significant role in regulating blood sugar levels and processing medications, making its health paramount to overall diabetes control.

While it can be easy to neglect, routine eye examinations by an ophthalmologist are essential to catch the early signs of diabetic retinopathy, a condition that can lead to blindness if not addressed posthaste.

Dental checks are another facet of health that can reflect the state of your diabetes management. Gum disease can be more prevalent and severe for those living with diabetes, so regular visits to the dentist help keep not only your mouth but also your blood sugar in check.

Your feet must not be forgotten in these regular health assessments. Neuropathy, or nerve damage, can cause a loss of feeling in your feet that might lead to infection or worse. Annual foot exams spot early signs of trouble while fostering discussions about proper foot care.

The cornerstone of diabetes management is not only in treatment but in prevention. Vaccinations like the flu shot and the pneumonia vaccine offer a shield of protection against illnesses that can complicate diabetes.

All these tests and check-ups provide valuable information but consider beyond the physical. These visits are opportunities to fortify the relationship with your healthcare team. Transparent conversations during these times can lead to critical adjustments in your diabetes management plan.

Embracing the rhythm of regular check-ups allows you to catch potential issues before they blossom into full-fledged problems. Like a diligent gardener who regularly checks for pests and diseases, you, too, must tend to the garden of your health with care and attention.

Remember, each test result is a snapshot, a moment in time. They do not define you but are tools to help you navigate the path of diabetes management with wisdom and care.

Participation in your health through these regular checkpoints reflects good stewardship of the body you've been given. As the passage of time brings change, these health markers are essential in revealing the true impact of your lifestyle choices on your diabetes.

Lastly, it's important to document and reflect upon the results from these check-ups. Keeping a record can illuminate patterns and progress, serving as encouragement and a cornerstone for a testimony of diligent management in the face of diabetes.

In conclusion, make regular check-ups and tests a priority. Regard them as invaluable touchpoints in your health's narrative and as an instrument to calibrate your care approach accurately. Let these consistent acts of maintenance reinforce your body's temple, allowing wellness to dwell richly within.

The Importance of Foot and Eye Care is a vital component in managing and thriving with type 2 diabetes. As we navigate this journey, we acknowledge that our bodies are temples, worthy of reverence and diligent care. The feet and eyes, in particular, require our utmost attention. They are, in many ways, the mirrors of our overall health, especially when living with diabetes.

Consider the feet: they are the foundation upon which we stand, integral to our mobility and independence. Yet, they are also highly vulnerable to complications due to diabetes. Neuropathy, a condition caused by elevated blood sugar levels damaging nerves over time, can lead to a loss of sensation in the feet. This numbness may prevent a person from feeling cuts or sores that can easily become infected. Moreover, poor circulation, another frequent challenge among those with diabetes, impedes the body's ability to heal, further elevating the risk of chronic wounds and even amputations. Thus, vigilant foot care is paramount—it's about preserving the very anatomical structures that allow us to walk in our purpose.

The friend that I mentioned earlier was affected hard by this one. He lost his foot, and then not too much later, he lost his leg at the knee due to diabetes. These are life altering changes and can be really tough to deal with for many. Proper foot care is essential for diabetics.

Setting a regular foot care regimen is a form of honoring the vessel given to us. Washing the feet daily with gentle soap and lukewarm water, diligently drying them to prevent fungal infections, and moisturizing to avoid cracked skin are all acts of worship in their own right. Regular self-examinations, akin to self-reflection, help spot the first signs of potential issues, and when done in partnership with healthcare professionals, it's a testament to the wise adage, "Faith without works is dead."

Like the feet, the eyes are a gift; they allow us to witness the beauty of creation, the faces of loved ones, and the world around us. Diabetes, however, can cast a shadow on this vision. Conditions such as diabetic retinopathy, where high blood sugar levels cause damage to the retina's blood vessels, can lead to severe vision loss if left unchecked. It's written, "Where there is no vision, the people perish," and so with diabetic eye care, we not only secure our physical sight but also our inner vision for a future filled with light and color.

Being proactive with eye care means scheduling regular comprehensive dilated eye exams—an act of preventative maintenance that ensures small issues can be identified and managed before they grow into mountains too tall to scale. Wearing sunglasses to shield against harmful ultraviolet rays, managing blood sugar levels meticulously, and maintaining blood pressure and cholesterol within healthy ranges, can be seen as armoring oneself in the full armor of righteousness.

In caring for our feet and eyes, we're reminded that our bodies are holistic entities, with each part connected to the greater whole. Just as the body of believers is diverse yet united, so too must our approach to health be integrative and cohesive. For instance, the footwear chosen must not only provide comfort and support but also protect the feet from injury. Similarly, nutritional choices that benefit overall health can directly improve eye health, highlighting the interconnectedness of our actions and their repercussions on our body's symphony.

Where much is given, much will be required. The responsibility of managing diabetes is significant, but it also brings with it the opportunity for growth and wisdom. Just as the wise man built his house upon the rock, so must we lay a strong foundation for our diabetes management on the bedrock of comprehensive foot and eye care. Prioritizing these aspects of health is not merely a practical concern but a spiritual mandate; for to see and walk in the path laid out for us, we must tend to the tools that make it possible.

Mindfulness in every step and glance can turn routine care into meditative practices. Each inspection of the feet, each appointment with the eye doctor, is a moment to pause, reflect, and give thanks for the body's wondrous capabilities, even as we work to preserve them.

It is in the mundane, everyday discipline of care that character is forged, and faith is lived out. Just as we are called to be faithful in the small things to be entrusted with larger things, so too with the daily act of foot and eye care—it is a sign of our stewardship over the physical temples entrusted to our care.

It's crucial to remember that while faith can move mountains, it is through our practical efforts that miracles of healing and restoration often manifest. The collaboration between divine faith and earthly wisdom found in diligent self-care is where true transformation unfolds. Therefore, it is not merely in the hope of health that we engage in foot and eye care, but in the active pursuit of it, with every tool and knowledge available to us.

Indeed, we walk by faith, not by sight, yet in caring for our sight and our ability to walk, we offer up a testimony of gratitude and reverence for the life we've been given. It's in these acts of care that we find the mundane transformed into the holy, as we maintain the health of our feet and the clarity of our eyesight.

So let us approach foot and eye care not as burdensome chores but as opportunities for reflection, gratitude, and ultimately, an expression of love—love for the Creator, love for ourselves as created beings, and love for the creation that we experience through our senses every day.

To pursue wellness through foot and eye care is to recognize that each day is a gift, and each mindful act of self-care is a means to honor that gift. In doing so, we embody a spirit of stewardship and respect for the intricate work of art that is the human body, a marvel of divine engineering.

Thus, foot and eye care become sanctified actions, avenues through which we engage with the world responsibly and respectfully. By focusing on these two critical aspects of self-care, we live out the calling to be caretakers of our bodies, never taking for granted the blessings of mobility and vision granted to us.

In conclusion, the importance of foot and eye care in diabetes management is both a practical necessity and a spiritual practice. It is an embodiment of the principle that to love oneself is the beginning of a lifelong romance. Nurturing our feet and eyes is a way of saying 'yes' to life, even amidst the trials of diabetes, holding fast to the conviction that we are fearfully and wonderfully made, with every step we take and every sight we behold.

Chapter 10:
Family, Friends, and Relationships

As we continue this journey together, let's acknowledge that our battles and triumphs aren't encountered in isolation. The fabric of our lives is intricately woven with the threads of connections to family, friends, and significant others. In acknowledging that 'no man is an island,' we begin to understand the mighty role that our relationships play in managing type 2 diabetes. Bonding with loved ones over shared challenges breeds resilience and inspiration. Educating those close to us not only empowers them to support us better but also embeds our commitment to health deep within our communal roots. From the simplest acts of modifying shared meals to promote wellness, to the complex dance of emotional support during vulnerable times, our connections can act as a scaffold, enhancing our strength to persevere and flourish. Throughout this chapter, we will explore the nuances of opening dialogues with our circle, the delicate balance of joy and health at social gatherings, and how to maintain intimacy and closeness when diabetes tries to claim a foothold. Anchored by the wisdom that "though one may be overpowered, two can defend themselves. A cord of three strands is not quickly broken," we are reminded that in unity, buoyancy can be found, allowing us to rise above the solitary struggle and engage in a harmonious chorus of support, engagement, and love.

Educating Your Loved Ones can seem daunting at first. It's reminiscent of tending a garden, nurturing the seedlings of understanding within the people you hold dear. A diagnosis of type 2 diabetes not only redirects your own life's course, but it also echoes through the lives of your family and friends. Just as you've embarked upon the journey of knowledge and adaptation, so too must they learn the twists and turns of this new path.

Let's begin with the foundation of empathy. Recall the parable of the sower, where seeds cast on good soil grow and flourish. Plant the seeds in the fertile ground of your loved ones' willingness to support you. Share your experiences with heartfelt honesty – express not only the practical aspects of diabetes management but also how this condition affects you emotionally and spiritually. Encourage them to walk this journey with you as partners in understanding.

Guidance starts at home. Anchor the education process in the serenity of your home environment, where questions can be asked and answered without the pressures of the outside world. Invite them to join you in meal planning and grocery shopping, turning these into opportunities to illuminate how dietary choices directly impact diabetes management. Participate jointly in preparing meals, underscoring the principles of a diabetes-friendly diet you've learned.

Equip your loved ones with the lifeboat of knowledge. Provide them with clear, simple-to-understand information about what type 2 diabetes entails. You might assemble a small pack with literature or direct them to reputable online resources. Also, consider inviting them to attend a diabetes education class with you. Learning side by side builds a shared understanding and brings a deeper appreciation for the small decisions that shape your well-being.

It's essential to also focus on the role of conversation. Engage in regular dialogue about your blood sugar levels and how various activities or foods affect them. This openness will not only reinforce your self-care routines but help your family and friends recognize patterns and offer meaningful support.

Understanding is bolstered in the forge of inquiry, so encourage your loved ones to ask questions. There can be a lot of misconceptions surrounding diabetes, and some may feel awkward or uneasy about broaching the subject. Make it clear that no question is too trivial or unwelcome, creating an atmosphere where curiosity leads to greater knowledge for everyone involved.

Include them in your sugar monitoring and medication routines. By allowing family and friends to witness or participate in these daily rituals, you demystify the process and educate them on why consistent monitoring and medication adherence are vital to your health.

When loved ones accompany you to medical appointments, they participate in the living narrative of your diabetes care. Here they can hear first-hand from healthcare professionals, ask their questions, and learn about the prognostic outlook directly, fostering a sense of inclusivity in your healthcare strategy.

Remember, too, that teaching is a two-way street. Your loved ones' perceptions and emotional responses hold insights that can strengthen your mutual support system. Listen to their concerns and feelings, acknowledging their important role in your journey. Doing so empowers them, turning passive concern into contributing action.

Patience is the key. Just as Moses led his people through the desert, you must guide your loved ones through the landscape of diabetes education. Some information might need repeating, and habits might take time to form. Celebrate the victories, no matter how small, and understand that setbacks are not failures but opportunities for reassessment and growth.

Use shared experiences to foster empathy and understanding. If opportunities arise for communities or church-based support groups for families dealing with diabetes, they can be invaluable. Connecting with others in similar situations widens the circle of support and provides alternative perspectives on common challenges.

Emphasize the connection between healthy living and spiritual well-being. When you tie the practice of caring for your body to the philosophy of nurturing the temple God has given you, it transcends the mere physical. This conceptual approach can resonate deeply, particularly with those who hold faith as an integral part of their lives.

Finally, ensure communication channels remain open and active. Whether it's through regular family meetings, emails, or messages in a shared family app, continual updates keep everyone informed and aligned with your needs and progress. It's like sending out regular epistles to your personal community, strengthening the network of care and concern around you.

In conclusion, educating your loved ones about your type 2 diabetes is not just about imparting knowledge; it's about building a community of care, a fellowship of understanding and support. As Proverbs 9:9 says, "Give instruction to a wise man, and he will be yet wiser: teach a just man, and he will increase in learning." Entrust in your collective wisdom to navigate through this together, with grace and fortitude.

Let this be but the initial steps in a shared odyssey of wellness and awareness. Continue to be a beacon of strength and knowledge for your loved ones, and let them be your sanctuary and support. For in this communion of education and care, you will find a deeper connection, not only managing your diabetes but enriching the bonds that tether you to those you love.

Navigating Social Gatherings and Holidays For those of us living with type 2 diabetes, the festive cheer of social gatherings and holidays can be a double-edged sword. These occasions offer a much-needed respite from our day-to-day routines and an opportunity to bond with loved ones, yet they often revolve around food and drink that can disrupt our carefully managed blood sugar levels. With thoughtful preparation and a heart filled with grace and understanding, we can still partake in these joyous events while maintaining our health and wellness.

The scripture offers wisdom in moderation, not just in sustenance but also in our actions. As Proverbs 25:16 says, "If you find honey, eat just enough— too much of it, and you will vomit." When approaching the laden tables of holiday feasts, take this wisdom to heart. Enjoy the tastes and pleasures of the food, but be mindful of portions. A small helping of your favorite dish can satisfy your soul without overtaxing your body.

Preparing for social gatherings may involve speaking with the host ahead of time. Communicate your dietary needs with humility and gratitude. Let your host know that while you are eager to participate, your health requires certain considerations. It's not about demanding special treatment, but about forging understanding. Most hosts will appreciate the heads-up and might make accommodations without a second thought.

Moreover, never forget the power in bringing your own contribution to the feast. Be it a diabetes-friendly dish or a sugar-free dessert, your offering doesn't just ease your own concerns but also introduces others to the delightful possibilities within diabetic nutrition. Sharing your journey through the foods you can enjoy opens the door for conversation and camaraderie.

When it comes to toasting and cheers, focus on spirit over spirits. Alcoholic beverages can have unpredictable effects on blood sugar and may not mix well with diabetes medications. If you do choose to partake, do so sparingly. There are also plenty of non-alcoholic options that can be just as festive. Celebratory doesn't have to mean inebriated. It means being present in the moment and savoring the connections.

During these occasions, routine may be your silent guardian. Checking blood sugar regularly becomes even more critical when your meal patterns fluctuate. It's easy to get caught up in the excitement and forget about monitoring, but those small discipline acts can guard you against potential highs and lows.

Exercise, too, can serve you well during these times. A morning walk or post-meal activity session can help mitigate the impact of a heavier-than-usual meal. Gather the family for a game of football or a brisk walk around the neighborhood. Not only does it help in managing your blood sugar, but it also creates beautiful memories and traditions.

When you're surrounded by scrumptious temptations, it's natural to feel deprived if you can't indulge as others do. However, refocus on the abundance already present in your life – the loved ones around you, the laughter shared, the unity felt. After all, these gatherings are less about the food and more about the people with whom you break bread.

And should you slip and indulge more than intended, be not harsh in self-judgment. Tomorrow brings another day for mindfulness and commitment. Guilt has no place at the table of self-care. Instead, learn from the experience and slowly steer back to your path with a renewed understanding of your triggers and temptations.

As the holidays approach, remember to safeguard your rest. Adequate sleep is paramount to maintaining your willpower and keeping stress levels, which can affect blood sugar, low. When we are tired, our body craves quick energy sources, often in the form of high sugar snacks – choosing rest is choosing strength.

In the heart of fellowship, individual strains become easier to bear, and support manifests in shared experiences. Initiating a conversation with a relative or friend who also manages diabetes can be enlightening. You may discover new strategies and feel bolstered knowing you're not navigating this journey alone.

Lastly, gratitude can be your sanctuary. Each meal shared, each laughter heard, is a testament to the life that flows within you and around you. Grace is realizing that diabetes is but a part of your journey, not the entirety of it. Be thankful for the knowledge you have to manage your condition and for the support you receive.

The passing of seasons is a reminder that life is indeed cyclical and full of change. Holidays and social gatherings will come and go, but the commitment to your well-being is an anchor that steadies you through it all. Lean on faith, embrace your knowledge, and walk forward with confidence. In this, find joy and the true essence of celebration.

So, when you next find yourself amidst a festive celebration or a holiday gathering, remember that you're not just navigating a diabetes-friendly path; you're cultivating balance, embracing love, and living life to its fullest. Let each gathering be a reflection of the beautiful tapestry of your life, vibrant threads of health, companionship, and joy woven together in harmony.

Diabetes and Sexuality Navigating the complex terrain of life with diabetes demands a comprehensive outlook, one that scrutinizes not just the physical aspects but also the interconnected nuances of one's entire being. Sexuality is a fundamental component of human health and well-being, a facet sometimes overshadowed by the pressing concerns of managing chronic conditions such as Type 2 diabetes. Yet, one cannot simply compartmentalize life into neat segments; the influence of diabetes stretches out, touching and often troubling the intimate waters of sexuality and relationships.

It is not uncommon for individuals with diabetes to encounter challenges in their sexual health. This could manifest in a multitude of ways for both men and women, ranging from physiological issues such as erectile dysfunction, vaginal dryness, or decreased libido, to psychological complexes rooted in self-image and emotional well-being. These are not just minor tribulations but significant concerns that can dampen the human spirit and crumble the bridges connecting souls in the most intimate manner.

The root of many sexual dysfunction issues rests, at least partially, in the complications brought forth by unregulated blood sugar levels. Elevated glucose can damage the vascular system and nerves, the very networks that are crucial for sexual arousal and response. Thus, rigorous blood sugar management becomes not only a pursuit for longevity and health but also for maintaining the vigor of one's intimate life. Always remember, your body is akin to a delicately woven tapestry; what affects one thread can compromise the integrity of the whole.

In the face of these challenges, take solace in the knowledge that you are not traversing this path alone. Countless individuals with diabetes have reclaimed the fullness of their sexuality through perseverance, openness, and strategic health management. The first step to addressing sexual dysfunction is to ignite the conversation with your healthcare provider. In these dialogues, find your voice and express your concerns without shame or fear; for truth spoken clears the mists of uncertainty and paves the way for healing.

Lifestyle modifications that you adopt to manage diabetes can also bolster sexual health. Regular exercise not only assists in glucose control but also enhances blood flow and energy levels, kindling the flames of desire and capacity. Likewise, a balanced diet—rich in nutrients and low in sugars and unhealthy fats—helps buoy your overall vitality and can lead to improved sexual function.

Medications for diabetes and other concurrent conditions may interfere with sexual function. These interactions are not merely coincidental but can be a direct consequence of the complex chemical ballet within your body. Do not hesitate to inquire about your treatment plan and its potential impact on your sexual health; adjustments can be made, and alternatives can be sought. It is written, "Ask and it shall be given to you," so ask with boldness and clarity.

Communication with your partner holds paramount importance in navigating the uncanny valley of diabetes and sexuality. It is through the mutual sharing of concerns and vulnerabilities that intimacy finds its deepest root and flourishes. Engage in open dialogues, not merely about the physical but about the emotional and spiritual—providing a sanctuary where love remains unshaken, even in the presence of adversity.

Mindfulness and stress management can be exceptional allies in your journey. Chronic stress can act as a vise upon your libido and sexual responsiveness. Integrate practices such as meditation, deep breathing exercises, or even therapeutic activities like art or music into your routine. These provide an oasis of tranquility in the bustling cityscape of life, allowing for rejuvenation of both body and soul.

For women, managing the hormonal fluctuations that affect blood sugar levels is a meticulous dance that requires attention. Embrace the counsel of specialists in women's health to bridge the gaps between endocrinological and gynecological aspects of diabetes care. In this mix, remember that your self-worth is not tethered to any physical condition or capacity but is an unalienable right born from the divine reflection within you.

For men, discussing sensitive issues such as erectile dysfunction with a healthcare professional can open doors to effective treatments, such as medication, devices, or counseling. It is not a sign of weakness to seek help but rather an act of courage; a step forward in faith, believing in the restoration of all good things.

Support groups and counseling can offer a communal salve for the emotional wounds that diabetes might inflict upon one's self-esteem and sense of sexuality. Sharing experiences, triumphs, and trials with others can dispel the clouds of isolation and affirm that love and companionship are not deficient but abound in abundance.

Couples may find it beneficial to work with a therapist or counselor familiar with the interplay between chronic illness and intimacy. These professionals can mold a space where exploration and growth occur, unfettered by judgment, illuminated by understanding, and graced with empathy—reflecting the belief that in our particular weaknesses, we find our most profound strength.

It is true that Type 2 diabetes can cast a long shadow, yet it need not reach into the sanctum of intimacy that you hold dear. Draw inspiration from the resilience that is a hallmark of the human spirit. The assurance found in committed partnership, the beauty in shared struggles, and the joy of overcoming each obstacle—these shine a light forward.

Celebrate small victories together with your partner, and remember that intimacy is born from more than physical connection; it is the union of minds, of hearts, of spirits walking in tandem along life's winding journey. Affirm each other, provide comfort, and never lose sight of hope, for it is the wellspring of life.

In summary, face diabetes with a holistic battle plan that includes safeguarding your sexuality. Embrace each day as an opportunity for connection, for love, and for renewal. As you venture through the landscape of life with diabetes, hold steadfastly to the conviction that you can experience a fulfilling, vibrant sexual life. This truth is as constant as the stars; your humanity, complete with its desires for intimacy and closeness, is a treasure to be cherished and pursued with grace and dignity.

Chapter 11:
The Financial Aspect of Diabetes Care

As we navigate the ever-winding path of managing diabetes, it's paramount to address the elephant in the room—the cost factor. Let's be candid: managing diabetes doesn't just demand your time and attention; it also requires a substantial financial commitment. However, fear not, for though the expenses may seem daunting at first, a beacon of hope shines bright. Understanding the inner workings of health insurance can illuminate avenues to alleviate the burden of medication costs. Embrace the practice of economical wisdom in your daily management; there are abundant budget-friendly tips and tricks specially designed to serve those striving on this journey. Take heart in knowing that, like the manna from heaven, there are assistance programs available, ready to provide succor to those in dire need. Remember, the investment you make today in your health is the foundation upon which a life filled with vibrancy and purpose is built—a life that is not defined by diabetes, but rather enriched by the triumph over its challenges.

Understanding Health Insurance and Medication Costs can often seem like navigating through a labyrinth, with various pathways offering different types of coverage and assistance. But don't be daunted; to lead a life tempered with grace and strength, one must understand how to manage and steward financial resources effectively, especially when it comes to health care for chronic conditions such as type 2 diabetes.

Health insurance for many is akin to a watchful shepherd, guiding and protecting the flock from the high costs of medical care. As someone with diabetes, it's essential to comprehend the full extent of your coverage. Your policy details what pharmaceuticals and treatments are covered and can significantly affect your out-of-pocket expenses.

Medication cost, in particular, deserves a closer look. It's important to discern between generic and brand-name drugs. Often, the generic version, which is scientifically equivalent to its brand-name counterpart, may be a fraction of the cost. Regularly reviewing your medication plan with your healthcare provider can ensure that your prescriptions are not only effective but also financially wise.

The intricacies of co-pays, deductibles, and out-of-network costs should be illuminated like verses from well-studied scripture. These terms dictate the shared cost between you and your insurance provider. A co-pay is a fixed amount you pay for a covered service, while a deductible is the amount you pay before your insurance starts to cover the costs. Understanding the stipulations of these payments can help you forecast your yearly diabetes care budget.

Furthermore, should you find your medication costs creeping higher than the mountains, it might be time to explore prescription assistance programs. Many pharmaceutical companies offer such programs, and they can be a boon to those who qualify, reducing the exorbitant costs to manageable streams of expenses.

Grasping the nuances of prior authorization can also prevent disruption in your treatment. Some insurers require that they pre-approve certain medications or procedures. Ensuring that this is in place is akin to seeking wisdom before making a decision – deliberate and prudent.

Insurance formularies are dynamic, akin to leaves in the wind, and so they change annually. These formularies are lists of drugs that insurers prefer and can impact what is affordable for you. Stay aware of these changes; a shift might mean that a medication you rely on suddenly becomes more expensive, or possibly that a more affordable option is available.

Navigating appeals processes can be like facing Goliath; daunting, yet not insurmountable. If your insurance denies coverage for a medication, know that you can appeal the decision. Thorough documentation and persistence are your slingshot and stones in such battles.

Also of note is the benefit design, which involves understanding the layout of your health plan. Does it offer a health savings account (HSA) or a flexible spending arrangement (FSA)? These pre-tax health funds can be like the loaves and fishes – seemingly limited, yet capable of stretching to meet your needs.

A word on Medicare and Medicaid: If these government programs are part of your coverage, it's crucial to understand the specific benefits and limitations. Each has different eligibility requirements and coverage specifics, but both can play a vital role in managing your medication costs. They serve as a lamp unto your financial pathway, guiding through the expenses of chronic care management.

Communication with your healthcare provider about cost is like seeking counsel; it is necessary for wise decision-making. Be open about your financial concerns. Physicians often know the cost-effective alternatives for treatments and can help you navigate through the options.

The Affordable Care Act has woven a safety net for many, with provisions such as prohibiting the denial of coverage due to pre-existing conditions. Explore insurance marketplaces to find a plan that aligns with your healthcare needs and financial ability. Remember, like a house upon a rock, a solid health plan is foundational to weathering the storm of chronic illness.

Lastly, do not overlook the support from your broader community. Non-profits and local organizations may offer additional resources and assistance. Their aid can be like manna in the wilderness, providing sustenance in times of need.

Remember, knowledge applied with discernment is wisdom, and wisdom in managing health insurance and medication costs is vital in your journey with diabetes. Equipped with understanding, you can be a steward of your health and advocate for your well-being, ensuring that while the body might be burdened with illness, the spirit thrives in the knowledge that you've taken control of your health care journey.

Thus, with courage and faith, approach the task of understanding your health insurance and medication costs. It is both a practical need and a profound opportunity to exercise wisdom, as you seek to live a full and abundant life with diabetes. It's about more than managing a disease; it's about nurturing the well-being of the body, mind, and spirit.

Budget-Friendly Tips for Managing Diabetes Managing diabetes needn't break the bank. Often, the journey through this condition can feel overwhelming, especially when figuring out how to care for your health, mindful of the expense. Yet, there are indeed strategies to navigate this path without incurring great cost, much like finding the way through wilderness guided by stars — it holds its own natural compass for those willing to seek it.

Finding affordable ways to manage diabetes aligns with the age-old wisdom that teaches us frugality and resourcefulness, virtues found in many a philosophical and biblical text. The key is to approach your diabetes management as a steward of your resources — both physical and financial.

To begin with, prioritize your grocery list to include whole, unprocessed foods. Vegetables and fruits that are in season, or even better, grown in your own garden, can be both fresher and cheaper. As the saying goes, "Give a man a fish, and you feed him for a day. Teach a man to fish, and you feed him for a lifetime." The act of growing your own food can be both spiritually rewarding and economically sensible.

When shopping, look out for sales and bulk-buy opportunities. Whole grains like brown rice, quinoa, and oats often come with a lower unit price in larger quantities. Store them properly, and they can serve as the basis for many a nutritious meal. As you make your loaves and fishes suffice, you'll discover how much can be saved.

Bargain hunting can also extend to your medication. Generic brands can be as effective as name brands, but come with a significantly lower cost. Consider speaking with your healthcare provider about the possibility of switching to a more affordable medication option. Much as the wisest of men sought value over price, so too should you seek the value in your treatment choices.

Another often-overlooked avenue of savings is prescription discount programs. These programs can reduce the cost of your medications significantly, especially if you are uninsured or your insurance does not cover certain prescriptions. "Ask and it shall be given to you," as the principle goes — inquire at your local pharmacy or do an online search for these programs.

Regular exercise is also a cornerstone of effective diabetes management and doesn't require expensive gym memberships. Walking, jogging, or cycling are all activities that are not only free but nurturing for the soul as well as the body. Remember, "The body is a temple," and as such, should be tended to with care and consistency.

Monitoring blood sugar doesn't have to be costly either. Some companies offer free meters if you buy their test strips, so it's worth doing some research. Furthermore, reach out to the diabetes community; often, others with diabetes might have tips on where to find supplies at a lower cost or may know of organizations that lend support.

Meal prepping is an effective strategy to both manage your diet and finances. Cooking in bulk can save both time and money, and as each meal is contained, so too is the temptation to indulge in foods that may not serve your health as well. "For what shall it profit a man, if he shall gain the whole world, and lose his own soul?" or, in this context, your health.

Keep a lookout for community events or local markets that offer health screenings and educational workshops at no cost. Knowledge is power, and building your understanding of diabetes can guide you to make informed decisions that are both cost-effective and beneficial to your health. As you nurture the seeds of wisdom, so too will you harvest health.

Don't dismiss the small lifestyle choices either. Take the stairs, use a basket instead of a cart at the grocery store, park further away from the entrance — each step is not only a step towards better health but a penny saved. Often, it's the small puddles of savings that can swell into a reservoir of resources.

Consider also peer support groups; fellowship can be as rich as any treasure. By sharing experiences and advice with others, you may find new ways to manage your diabetes that are more cost-effective or efficient. Such camaraderie on your journey can be uplifting, lessening the burden on both your spirit and wallet.

Lastly, keep in mind that while cutting costs is important, investing in your health will always yield high returns. Take care not to skimp on necessary supplies or treatments for the sake of saving money. Your health is invaluable, and remembering this is crucial as you navigate the financial aspects of diabetes care.

Remember, managing your diabetes with financial astuteness is not only about spending less but spending wisely. It is about understanding that each penny saved with intelligence is akin to the parable of the talents — it is an investment in the health and wealth of your life.

In sum, managing diabetes within a modest budget is an attainable and rewarding endeavor. Like the faith that moves mountains, you'll find that a faith in your own ability to manage diabetes resourcefully can transform mountains of expense into manageable hills. With steadfast determination and prudent practice, you'll find peace and strength along this journey of managing diabetes.

Accessing Assistance Programs and Resources As we journey along the path of managing diabetes, we often find ourselves at intersections where guidance is much needed. This guidance may come in the form of assistance programs and resources specifically designed to lend a hand to those who are navigating the intricacies of life with type 2 diabetes. Walking this path requires knowledge not only of the physical and emotional aspects of the condition but also of the practical support available to us.

Navigating the healthcare system can be likened to seeking light through a dense forest. Assistance programs act as beams of light, providing financial aid, medication discounts, or educational resources. Each individual's path is unique, and as such, the search for assistance must be tailored to one's own needs. The first step is recognizing that seeking help is an act of wisdom and strength rather than a sign of weakness.

In the Scriptures, asking for help is seen as an act of faith, and similarly, we must put faith in the systems designed to support us. Local government and non-profit organizations often run programs that assist with the cost of medication, supplies like blood glucose testing strips, and nutritional advice. Start by contacting your local health department to inquire about available diabetes support programs.

Moreover, pharmaceutical companies sometimes offer assistance programs for medications. These Patient Assistance Programs (PAPs) could significantly reduce or even eliminate the cost of your diabetes medication. To find out if you are eligible for such programs, a visit to the drug manufacturer's website or a conversation with your healthcare provider can set you on the right path.

Insurance plans can be a maze of complexity, but understanding your coverage is critical. In-depth conversations with your insurance provider about specific diabetes management coverage can illuminate benefits you might not be aware of, such as coverage for nutritionist consultations or educational workshops. Don't hesitate to ask for a review of your plan; the representatives are there to serve as your torchbearers.

Community health clinics are also a wellspring of support, offering sliding-scale services based on income. They may provide affordable access to healthcare providers, education, and even discounted medications and supplies. They are a testament to the community spirit, where helping one another is a central tenet.

For those who are eligible, Medicare and Medicaid can be valuable resources. They offer coverage that may include diabetes education, nutritional services, and diabetes-related medical supplies. Investigating these governmental programs can take time, but they can provide a financial cushion for your healthcare needs.

Nutrition is foundational in managing diabetes, and various organizations offer meal assistance programs. These include services such as home-delivered meals tailored for diabetes or programs like Supplemental Nutrition Assistance Program (SNAP), which can help increase your access to healthy foods. As the bread of life sustains us spiritually, so does proper nutrition sustain our bodies.

The internet is an unparalleled resource for diabetes education. From understanding the nuances of your condition to learning self-care practices, numerous reputable websites and online communities are at your fingertips. Don't underestimate the value of these communal wells of knowledge, for they are a gathering of minds and experiences that can enrich your understanding.

Faith-based organizations may also offer assistance for those with diabetes. These groups can provide not only spiritual support but also physical donations of supplies or services. Connecting with your local place of worship can open doors to compassionate assistance aligned with your faith journey.

Prescription discount cards and programs can serve as financial manna, offering reduced prices for medications. While these programs may not lower costs as much as insurance or PAPs, they can still ease the burden for those who are uninsured or underinsured. Compare different programs to see which offers the best benefits for your specific medicinal needs.

For the working individual, the Americans with Disabilities Act (ADA) is a protective shield. It ensures that employers provide reasonable accommodations for employees with diabetes. Understanding your rights under the ADA can empower you to maintain both your health and your livelihood.

When exploring assistance programs, organization is paramount. Keep detailed records of all your healthcare expenses, medications, and insurance. A well-maintained log serves as a roadmap, helping you and those assisting you to make informed decisions about which programs you can benefit from.

Remember, the early bird catches the worm when it comes to assistance programs. Many have limited funding and are served on a first-come, first-served basis. Timely action and perseverance are vital in securing the support you need.

Finally, remember that you're not alone on this pilgrimage. There are healthcare professionals, patient advocates, and diabetes educators whose vocation is to assist you. Reach out to them, ask questions, and learn about new services and programs that could ease your journey.

Embarking on the quest for assistance requires both courage and humility, reflecting the biblical principle that in our weakness, we find strength. We're faced with the duality of acknowledging our need for help, while also embracing the self-advocacy required to pursue it. In every season, be it a valley or mountaintop, seek the available resources with optimism and a proactive spirit. Together, let us build a bridge to a healthier, more supported life with diabetes.

Chapter 12:
Innovations in Diabetes Care

As we journey through the landscape of managing Type 2 diabetes, the horizon is changing, revealing a sun that sets with hope for a transformed tomorrow. Continuous streams of innovation quench the thirst for easier, more effective routes to wellness, flourishing as tools and treatments capable of rewriting the narrative of diabetes care. The painstaking effort invested in the past paves the way for new possibilities—the latest technologies become lanterns in the night, guiding us along a previously dim path. From monitoring blood glucose levels without a single drop of blood to encapsulated pancreas cells aiming to restore natural insulin function, these strides signify a bountiful promise—one of less pain, greater accuracy, and unwavering support. At times, the progress may seem like a creeping vine, slow to cover the imposing walls of chronic illness, but each advancement carries with it the potential to change lives profoundly. Embrace the innovative spirit of this era and consider contributing to the cure by participating in clinical trials—your invaluable contribution could lead you to become part of a legacy that turns the tide in the battle against diabetes.

The Latest in Diabetes Technology As we turn the page on the traditional methods of diabetes management, we find ourselves stepping into a new era marked by groundbreaking technological innovations. These advances, harnessing the power of the digital age, offer not just convenience and precision but also a sense of empowerment in the management of type 2 diabetes.

Continuous glucose monitoring (CGM) systems have revolutionized how individuals with diabetes track and manage their blood glucose levels. Gone are the days of frequent finger pricks and blood samples. CGM devices now provide real-time glucose readings throughout the day and night, revealing trends and allowing for immediate response to prevent potential highs and lows.

The inspired integration of smart insulin pens into the diabetes management repertoire has been a game changer. For those who may not be on pump therapy, these smart pens offer dosing calculators, reminders, and the ability to sync with other digital devices, ensuring dosages are accurate and adherence to treatment plans is meticulously recorded.

Insulin pump technology itself has seen impressive advancements. Modern pumps not only deliver insulin but also communicate with CGM systems for a more closed-loop system, taking proactive steps in adjusting insulin delivery based on glucose readings—a stride towards the artificial pancreas.

Furthermore, diabetes management apps have filled our smartphones with their beneficial presence. It's as though one has a medical advisor in their pocket, providing insights on dietary choices, medication reminders, and activity suggestions personalized to their unique health profile.

Telemedicine, a beacon of modern healthcare, has come to the forefront, particularly highlighted during the challenges of recent times. Now, one can consult with healthcare professionals from the comfort of their home, facilitating regular check-ups and garnering expert advice without the barriers of travel and time.

Advances in the realm of medical data analytics provide a new understanding gleaned from the vast seas of personal health data collected over time. This data, when synthesized, offers custom predictions and advice, guiding individuals on a path towards optimal health outcomes with unprecedented personalization.

Even the supporting accessories of diabetes management have evolved. The design and functions of carrying cases for insulin and other diabetes supplies now embody a seamless blend of style, security, and temperature-controlled environments, assuring one's supplies are both discreet and in prime condition.

Nutritional technology has also taken leaps forward, with flash glucose monitoring devices providing immediate analysis of food intake against current glucose levels, furnishing instantaneous feedback to enhance dietary decision-making.

At the heart of these technological strides lies the power of community. Online platforms bring together those on the diabetes journey, facilitating the exchange of stories, tips, and support. This digital companionship fosters a collective strength that transcends geographical boundaries.

Moreover, research in predictive analytics and artificial intelligence creates a proactive approach in diabetes management. These technologies are beginning to offer a glimpse of tomorrow where potential episodes of hypoglycemia or hyperglycemia might be anticipated and preemptively managed.

Stemming from these innovations, there is nascent research looking into smart tattoos. These tattoos aim to change color based on glucose levels in the interstitial fluid. Imagine a future where one's own skin anchors an intrinsic glucose monitoring system, artfully intertwining functionality with the canvas of the body.

Yet, with all these technological advancements, it is vital to remember the importance of the human element. Technology serves as a tool to enhance, not replace, the wisdom and nurturing care of healthcare providers. It complements the invaluable support from family, friends, and the diabetes community.

And in this convergence of science and human touch, there's an echo of something greater, an undercurrent that reminds us of the intricate design of our bodies and the profound resilience within. It's as if each technological breakthrough mirrors the precision and capability infused within creation, reminding us of the balance one must navigate between the material and the spiritual.

In embracing these latest technologies, one not only adapts to the present landscape of diabetes management but also becomes a participant in shaping the future. Each innovation adopted, each shared experience, contributes to the collective wisdom that paves the way for what lies beyond the horizon.

Leveraging the promise offered by these advancements in technology, one can journey forward with confidence, knowing that the voyage is embraced with tools that illuminate the path. As we look towards the emergent wonders of diabetes care, let's contemplate the potential they hold to transform mere management into a symphony of synchronized, seamless living with type 2 diabetes.

Future Treatments on the Horizon In the ever-forward march of medical progress, there is light that flickers on the horizon—a beacon of hope for those living with type 2 diabetes. As we have traversed the landscape of understanding this condition and adapting our lives to manage it well, let us lift our eyes to the advancements that lie ahead. It is in these potential future treatments that we begin to see the silhouette of breakthrough, the promise of easier days, and the possibility of renewed health.

Researchers are working tirelessly, not just to improve the quality of care, but also to discover revolutionary treatments that could alter the course of diabetes management. Imagine a world where the daily routines of finger-pricking and meticulous diet tracking are eased by new innovations. This is not a mere daydream but a potential reality as science delves deeper into understanding how our bodies work and how they can be encouraged to heal themselves.

One avenue of exploration focuses on the regeneration of beta cells—the very cells in our pancreas responsible for producing insulin. Through the development of drugs that promote beta cell growth, the body's natural ability to regulate blood sugar levels could be restored, reducing the need for external insulin. Such advancements wouldn't just change treatment modalities; they would transform lives.

There is also growing attention on the power of microbiome therapy. As the scientific community becomes more acquainted with the profound influence of gut bacteria on overall health, there's mounting evidence that rebalancing these microscopic communities could benefit those with diabetes. Modifying the microbiome might improve insulin sensitivity and glucose metabolism, creating a more harmonious internal environment.

On the wings of technological innovation, researchers are painting the picture of smart insulin—insulin that would be activated only when needed. This exceptional concept involves insulin that would circulate in the bloodstream in an inactive form and would only switch "on" when blood glucose levels rise. After normalizing sugar levels, it would seamlessly return to its inert state. This smart insulin could one day eliminate the fear of hypoglycemia and dramatically simplify diabetes management.

Gene therapy also stands on the periphery, gearing up to make its grand entrance into the diabetes arena. With the goal of correcting or replacing the genetic mutations that can lead to diabetes, gene therapy looms as a pivotal chapter in our story of triumph over chronic illness. Such a fundamental approach has the potential to mend the root causes of diabetes, rather than merely tempering its symptoms.

Contributing to these innovations are advancements in nanotechnology. Consider particles so small they can navigate our bloodstream and deliver medications directly to target cells. These microscopic couriers are being developed to improve the efficacy and precision of diabetes medications, lowering the risk of side effects and improving outcomes.

Artificial pancreas systems, which would take automation a step further than current insulin pumps and continuous glucose monitors, are under development. These systems aim to replicate the glucose-regulating function of a healthy pancreas, automatically adjusting insulin delivery based on real-time changes in blood sugar levels, activity, and the individual's physiological needs.

Immunotherapy represents another beacon of innovation. This approach seeks to temper the immune system's errant assault on pancreatic cells, retraining the body's defenses to restore harmony within. In cases of type 2 diabetes, where inflammation and an overactive immune response play a role, immunotherapy holds the promise of re-establishing balance.

Let us also turn our gaze to the potential of personalized medicine. As each individual's journey with diabetes is unique, the ability to tailor treatments based on genetic, lifestyle, and environmental factors could usher in a new era of customized care. This approach would represent a seismic shift from the one-size-fits-all model to one where your treatment is as unique as you are.

Moreover, the promise of new oral medications that would not only manage glucose levels but also address other related health concerns, such as cardiovascular disease, is on the rise. These dual-function medications could become the cornerstone of a more comprehensive approach to treating type 2 diabetes, looking beyond blood sugar control alone.

Stem cell therapy, one of the most anticipated fields of study, is on a path that might redefine the very fabric of diabetes treatment. The ability to create insulin-producing cells from stem cells and transplant them into people with diabetes could offer a reprieve from the unceasing demands of the condition. The pursuit of this therapy brings us closer to the day when replenishing insulin may no longer require an external source.

Not to be overlooked is the expansion of wearable technology beyond current glucose monitoring systems. Future devices could provide real-time insights into a wider range of health metrics, offering comprehensive health monitoring and actionable data that could prevent complications before they begin.

Furthermore, research into dietary supplements and herbal medicines continues to evolve. Unveiling the potential of natural compounds to support better blood sugar control, these treatments could one day be integrated into the standardized regimen for managing diabetes, bridging the gap between traditional wisdom and modern medicine.

As we look to the future with optimism, it's important to remember that our journey with diabetes is a voyage of personal discovery and adaptation. While we eagerly anticipate the arrival of new treatments, it is up to us to maintain our health with the tools currently at our disposal. The promise of tomorrow shines brightly, inspiring us to persevere today. With faith as our compass and hope as our anchor, we can navigate the challenges of diabetes, anticipating the day when these future treatments render the burden of this condition a distant memory.

Participating in Clinical Trials As individuals grapple with the realities of living with type 2 diabetes, it's not uncommon to seek new avenues for treatment and management of the condition. Participating in clinical trials is one such avenue that not only provides access to cutting-edge therapies but also contributes to the greater good of advancing medical knowledge and helping future generations. In the spirit of seeking out new landscapes for healing, let's delve into the realm of clinical trials specifically designed for those with type 2 diabetes.

Clinical trials are research studies that explore whether a medical strategy, treatment, or device is safe and effective for humans. These studies also may show which medical approaches work best for certain illnesses or groups of people. It's an opportunity for participants to play a proactive role in their care, receiving close monitoring by healthcare professionals and access to treatments that are not yet widely available.

The design of these trials is typically rigorous, often involving several phases that test a treatment's safety, effectiveness, and side effects. It's like embarking on a meticulously planned journey, each step building upon the last to reach a pinnacle of understanding that can bless the lives afflicted by this challenging condition.

Venturing into a clinical trial is a leap of faith, akin to the faith of David facing Goliath, relying not on conventional arms, but on the power of innovation and the spirit of discovery. For those managing diabetes, it's a testament to strength, participating in a trial means entrusting your health to medical researchers and contributing to a lineage of clinical advancements.

One might wonder, why consider joining a trial? The opportunity to access new treatments that could be more effective than existing ones can be a beacon of hope for those who feel that their current management plan is lacking. Participants are closely monitored, and this can bring a reassuring level of checking and balancing one's health, echoing the vigilant shepherding of one's body.

Enrolling in a trial typically begins with a process called informed consent. This is a fundamental right, akin to wise counsel, and a crucial step ensuring that participants are aware of the potential risks and benefits, much as one would count the cost before building a tower. This process exemplifies the principle of walking into a situation with one's eyes wide open, making decisions in consciousness rather than in ignorance.

It's essential to converse with healthcare providers before enrolling in a clinical trial. They can offer guidance and discernment, much as Solomon used wisdom to govern his decisions. Providers can help assess whether the trial's focus aligns well with one's individual health needs and goals. It's a collaborative consultation that can pave the way for a fruitful journey through the trial.

Eligibility is another cornerstone of clinical trial participation. Each study has criteria that need to be met, which may include age, gender, the type and stage of diabetes, previous treatment history, and other medical conditions. Reflect upon the story of Esther, who found herself uniquely positioned for the role she needed to play. Similarly, the specific circumstances of one's health may align perfectly with a trial's requirements.

Throughout participation in a clinical trial, the spirit of stewardship must prevail. It is crucial to take responsibility for understanding the commitments involved, from the frequency of study visits to the procedures and treatments one will undergo. Like a steward tending to a vineyard, attention and care to these details bear the fruit of a well-managed trial experience.

Many trials are blinded or placebo-controlled, meaning participants may not know if they are receiving the active treatment or a placebo. This process can be thought of as walking by faith, not by sight, trusting in the structured methods of the study, aiming to preserve the validity of the results, and ultimately benefit the broader community.

Consider the possible side effects and interventions. They are part of the landscape in this exploration of uncharted territories. Just as every valley has its lilies and every mountain its hardships, it is wise to prepare for adversities, recognizing that every step in a trial is aimed toward reaching a higher ground in diabetes treatment.

Participation in a clinical trial is not without its uncertainties but offers the peace that comes from being at the frontline of potential breakthroughs. It's a peace akin to that found in the midst of a storm, knowing that even the challenges faced can lead to a path of progress for oneself and others who travel the same road.

The conclusion of a trial does not necessarily mean instant results. Patience is akin to farmers waiting for their fields: each season brings its harvest in due time. Data must be gathered, analyzed, and reviewed, and treatments must pass through regulatory approval before they can be accessible to the greater public. Participants in clinical trials are like sowers of seeds, which may bloom long after the initial planting.

Engaging with others who have walked this path can be a source of inspiration and practical wisdom. Testimonials can be likened to parables, teaching through personal anecdotes and shared experiences. They offer the insight and encouragement that can reinforce the decision to embark on the trial or provide comfort during challenging moments within the journey.

In conclusion, participating in clinical trials is a bridge between the known and the unknown, representing hope, courage, and commitment to progress in the realm of type 2 diabetes. Much like the faith that moves mountains, persistence in research can lead to breakthroughs that shift the current paradigms of diabetes care. For those considering this path, it is a noble endeavor, holding promise for oneself and the future of many.

Chapter 13:
Thriving with Diabetes

The journey you have embarked upon, one with Type 2 Diabetes, is undeniably laden with challenges, adjustments, and learning curves. The tapestry of life, however, remains rich and vibrant, its threads woven with perseverance and hope. And in this concluding chapter, we gather the wisdom from previous pages to reinforce the idea that not only can one live with diabetes, but one can indeed thrive.

When informed of your diagnosis, it might have seemed like a daunting mountain to climb. Yet, through embracing your nutritional blueprint, discovering the empowering effects of exercise, and understanding the intricacies of medication and monitoring, you are already ascending towards a summit of well-being. Life, as it unfolds with diabetes, can be full of moments both ripe with vitality and reflective in nature.

In this management of blood sugars and careful balance of daily habits, there is a profound lesson akin to the philosophical and biblical teachings that have guided humankind for ages. It is the lesson of mastery over the body – not as a harsh ruler, but as a wise and understanding steward. Your body is a temple, a trusted vessel, and by listening and responding to it with care, you honor the gift of life bestowed upon you.

We have discussed the significance of nourishment – not just physical, but mental and emotional as well. Just as important as the food that fuels your body is the positive mindset that propels your spirit. The narratives of defeat are replaced with liturgies of triumph. You shoulder the diagnosis with dignity, viewing it not as a life sentence, but as a call to live mindfully and passionately.

Your path will be unique, as no two individuals with diabetes will have identical experiences. What remains consistent, though, is the ability to exert control, to make choices that favor vitality over complacency. Every healthy meal, every burst of activity, and every night of restorative sleep is a victory, a building block in the fortress against complications.

As you've navigated the practicalities of day-to-day life with diabetes, from managing the highs and lows to traveling and dealing with sick days, you have gained invaluable skills. These skills extend beyond the management of a condition; they fortify your ability to adapt, to be resilient, and to thrive in circumstances that once seemed overwhelming.

Mindfulness is integral to this thriving. It roots you in the present moment, allowing for the acknowledgement of emotions, the savoring of life's small pleasures, and the acceptance of what is beyond one's control. Embrace the stillness and wisdom found in the 'now', letting go of the burdens of yesterday and the anxieties of tomorrow.

Your relationships, too, play a pivotal role in your well-being. Educating loved ones, navigating social gatherings, and maintaining intimacy are testaments to the depth and strength of your connections. These bonds provide sustenance just as vital as any nutrient-dense meal, enriching your life with love and support.

The intersecting of the financial aspect of diabetes care with your life's tapestry is undeniable. Yet, by demystifying health insurance, adapting with budget-friendly tips, and accessing resources, you transform what could be an overwhelming burden into another aspect of life you confidently manage. With every prudent financial choice, you invest in your longevity and quality of life.

Take heart in recognizing the astonishing innovations in diabetes care. From the advancements in technology to promising future treatments and the potential found in clinical trials, there is a sea of opportunity on the horizon. These developments are not merely medical breakthroughs; they are beacons of hope, signaling an even brighter future for all living with diabetes.

Thriving transcends mere survival; it requires an affirmative choice, a daily decision to seek joy, nurture your body, expand your mind, and envelop your spirit with peace. As you continue to live with diabetes, may you draw strength not just from practical knowledge, but from the enduring truth that every day brings the chance for new growth and fresh beginnings.

There will be moments of difficulty, times when the smooth sailing of life's journey is replaced by stormy seas. In those moments, remember the profound strength you have cultivated, the wisdom you have accumulated, and the unceasing support that surrounds you. You are not a solitary traveler but a vital part of a community, a tapestry of lives interconnected through shared experiences and aspirations.

Your story is not merely one of managing a condition; it is an epic penned with courage, a narrative of overcoming and becoming – becoming more than you ever thought possible. In the silent whispers of your heart and the jubilant celebrations of your achievements, may you always find the melody of a life lived fully and fearlessly.

As we bring this guide to a close, remember that living with Type 2 Diabetes is not the dimming of a light, but a call to shine brighter. It is not the end of a journey, but an opportunity to tread a path dappled with wisdom, resourcefulness, and hope. Take each step forward with confidence, for you are equipped, you are capable, and you are never alone.

Therefore, let us not see diabetes as a storm cloud that casts a shadow over our days, but rather as a catalyst that urges us to seek out the colors of the rainbow that emerge thereafter. And so, embrace the life you have been given, with all its unique challenges and blessings. Empowered with knowledge, surrounded by love, and upheld by faith, go forth and thrive, for this is not just a possibility – it is your destined reality.

Appendix A:
Diabetes-Friendly Recipes and Snacks

As we journey through the various facets of living with type 2 diabetes, we recognize that nourishment plays a central role not merely in sustaining life but in enhancing its quality. Our bodies are temples, deserving of care and respect. With every bite, we have the opportunity to honor our bodies, cater to our needs, and uplift our spirits. The recipes and snacks included here are not only friendly to your diabetic lifestyle but are designed to bring joy to your palate and vigor to your body.

In this collection, you'll find dishes that weave together the goodness of whole, unprocessed ingredients with the aromatic spices and herbs that elevate both flavor and health benefits. These recipes are not just about keeping blood sugar levels within the desired range; they're about creating moments of delight at your dining table. Living with diabetes doesn't mean forsaking delicious meals—it's about discovering new ways to savor every meal.

Breakfasts to Kickstart Your Day

Wholesome Oat and Chia Porridge with Berries

Scrambled Egg Whites with Spinach and Mushrooms

Almond Flour Pancakes Topped with a Cinnamon-Apple Compote

Nourishing Main Courses

Grilled Lemon-Herb Chicken with Quinoa Pilaf

Zucchini Noodles Tossed in a Roasted Garlic and Tomato Sauce

Spiced Lentil Stew with Brown Rice

Hearty Salads and Sides

Kale and Avocado Salad with a Sprinkling of Sunflower Seeds

Roasted Brussels Sprouts with a Balsamic Glaze

Cauliflower Rice Seasoned with Turmeric and Coriander

Snacks for Sustained Energy

Carrots and Hummus Dip

Apple Slices with Almond Butter

Homemade Trail Mix with Nuts and Unsweetened Dried Fruit

Revitalizing Beverages

Green Smoothie with Spinach, Avocado, and Chia Seeds

Herbal Tea Infusions like Chamomile or Peppermint

Chilled Cucumber-Mint Water

Each of these recipes understands the tapestry of needs for those managing type 2 diabetes. You'll find that the ingredients are high in nutrients, fiber-rich, and possess a low glycemic index to ensure a modest impact on blood sugar. However, their value lies not solely in their nutritional profile but in their capacity to heal and comfort the body like a warm, welcoming home, and to satisfy the soul like a lush garden of delights.

Through these culinary creations, the endeavor is not just to feed the needs of the body but also to nourish the heart and renew the spirit. They're designed to give you a sense of empowerment and joy, sure to inspire smiles at your table. Remember, variety is the spice of life, and integrating these diverse dishes into your routine will not only uphold your nutritional needs but will also provide a canvas for creativity and discovery in your own kitchen.

There's a profound beauty in the simplicity of a meal prepared with care and intention. These recipes embody that sentiment—they are invitations to taste the abundance of the earth, mindful of the body's requirements and the heart's yearnings. As you partake in these meals, may they be a source of pleasure and health, and may your journey with diabetes be one filled with many such gratifying and life-affirming moments. You will be able to find more diabetic friendly recipes and cookbooks on my corporate website at www.MyMaverickWorld.com.

Appendix B:
Exercise Logs and Food Diaries

Maintaining a record of your physical activity and dietary intake is not merely a task; it is a profound strategy, a form of stewardship over the temple that is your body. We've journeyed through the mechanics of managing diabetes, and now we've reached an essential tool in your arsenal—the art of tracking. In these logs and diaries, the story of your progress is penned, revealing patterns and truths that may otherwise remain unseen.

Why Keep an Exercise Log?

An exercise log serves as a mirror reflecting the efforts you pour into your well-being. It isn't just about marking down minutes and movements; it's about recognizing your daily victories, no matter their size. Recording your exercises helps you to:

Ensure consistency and progression in your workout routine.

Identify what types of exercise resonate with your body and soul.

Map out how your body responds to physical activity over time.

Celebrate milestones that might otherwise go unnoticed.

Resist the temptation to see exercise as a burden; rather, see it as a blessing, an opportunity for renewal.

How to Maintain an Effective Food Diary

Similarly, a food diary is more than a log; it is a testament of nourishment, an acknowledgment of every choice that sustains your life. With each entry, you're invited to:

Monitor your nutritional intake to balance carbohydrates, proteins, and fats.

Recognize triggers for glucose spikes and identify foods that stabilize your levels.

Understand your eating patterns and how they align with your emotions and activities.

Discern moderation and adjust portions to align with your health goals.

As it is written, "Man does not live by bread alone," and your food diary encompasses the entirety of what it means to feed oneself with intention and mindfulness.

Getting Started

Begin your exercise and food diary by considering simplicity and sustainability. Choose a means that resonates with your lifestyle, be it a written journal, a smartphone app, or a spreadsheet. Remember this: the value of your logs lies not in their complexity, but in their honest reflection of your daily journey.

Select a method for tracking that you'll consistently use.

Set aside dedicated time each day for inputting your exercise and food data.

Be as detailed as possible with the types of foods, portion sizes, and exercise specifics, including duration and intensity.

Observe trends and use them to inform your ongoing decisions about food and exercise.

In the quiet moments when you review your logs, let there be a spirit of gratitude—for the body that allows you to move, for the food that fuels you, for the choice to care for yourself. Let each entry be a stepping stone on your path to wellness, a tangible manifestation of the unwavering commitment to your health. Walk this path with intention, knowing that with each step, you are forging a better tomorrow.

Appendix C:
Resource Directory for Diabetes Support

As we journey through life with diabetes, we discover that support comes in many forms. It's the comforting voice at the end of a helpline, the rich pool of knowledge from books and websites, and the fellowship found in support groups. This resource directory for diabetes support is curated to uplift and sustain you on your path.

National Diabetes Organizations

American Diabetes Association (ADA): Offers comprehensive information on diabetes care, local support groups, and advocacy efforts. Visit *diabetes.org* to learn more.

Centers for Disease Control and Prevention (CDC) - Diabetes Home: Provides a wealth of public health information and resources on diabetes. Their site is *cdc.gov/diabetes*.

National Institute of Diabetes and Digestive and Kidney Diseases (NIDDK): Supports research and education on diabetes. Their resources can be accessed at *niddk.nih.gov*.

Educational Resources

Diabetes Self-Management Education and Support (DSMES) services: Enhance your skills and knowledge to live well with diabetes. Locate an accredited DSMES program on *diabeteseducator.org*.

Mayo Clinic - Diabetes: Offers expert advice and information on managing diabetes from renowned healthcare professionals at *mayoclinic.org/diseases-conditions/diabetes*.

Online Support Groups and Forums

Fostering connections with individuals who understand your experiences can foster hope and resilience. Explore these online communities for shared stories and support:

Diabetes Daily: Join discussions and access educational materials at *diabetesdaily.com*.

dLife Community: Connect with others, ask questions, and share your journey on *dLife.com*.

Health and Wellness

Nurturing your body, mind, and spirit plays a significant role in managing diabetes:

SparkPeople: Discover diabetes-friendly recipes and workout tips on *sparkpeople.com*.

Mindful Diabetic: Engage with resources focused on the holistic aspect of diabetes care at *mindfuldiabetic.com*.

Faith-Based Support

Faith can serve as a pillar of strength in times of uncertainty. Seek out local faith communities with health ministries or explore online resources like:

Faith & Diabetes: A platform for integrating faith-based practices in diabetes management. Visit *faithanddiabetes.org* for more information.

Remember, the support you seek as you manage your diabetes can illuminate the path ahead with wisdom and compassion. Each resource you tap into is like a beacon, casting light on your journey and empowering you to live your fullest life. As it has been said, "Two are better than one, because they have a good return for their labor: If either of them falls down, one can help the other up." (Ecclesiastes 4:9-10a). Embrace the community and expertise that surround you, and let them guide you towards vitality and wellness.

Glossary of Diabetes Terms

As we journey together through the valleys and peaks of managing diabetes, knowledge becomes our lantern, illuminating the path towards a life well-lived. The terms listed below serve as signposts, directing us towards understanding and empowerment.

A1C

A1C: A test that reflects average blood glucose levels over the past 2-3 months, providing insight into overall glucose control. Think of it as the "big picture" in your diabetes management canvas.

Basal Insulin

Basal Insulin: The insulin that's required to manage blood sugar levels in a fasting state or between meals. It's like the constant hum of a lighthouse, keeping things steady through the night.

Blood Glucose Monitor

Blood Glucose Monitor: A device used to measure the concentration of glucose in the blood, a compass in the hands of the traveler.

Carbohydrate Counting

Carbohydrate Counting: A method of meal planning where carbs are tracked to manage blood sugar levels. It invites mindfulness and intention into each meal, much like selecting stones to build a steadfast foundation.

Diabetes Self-Management Education (DSME)

Diabetes Self-Management Education (DSME): Structured education that equips individuals with the skills needed to cope with diabetes and care for their health. Consider it wisdom passed down, a wellspring of knowledge to draw from.

Endocrinologist

Endocrinologist: A doctor specializing in the endocrine system, including diabetes. They guide explorers through the intricate interplay of hormones and health.

Fasting Plasma Glucose

Fasting Plasma Glucose (FPG): A test to measure blood sugar levels after an eight-hour fast, providing an assessment of the body's glucose maintenance capabilities.

Glycemic Index

Glycemic Index (GI): A ranking of foods based on their immediate effect on blood glucose levels. It's akin to understanding the nature of the ground beneath one's feet—some terrain will slow you down, while other ground lets you traverse quickly.

Hyperglycemia

Hyperglycemia: A condition characterized by higher than normal blood sugar levels. It's a warning signal, much like a storm on the horizon, urging action to restore balance.

Hypoglycemia

Hypoglycemia: A condition where blood sugar levels drop below normal. It compels immediate attention like a shepherd tending to a wayward lamb.

Insulin Pump

Insulin Pump: A small, portable device that delivers insulin through the body throughout the day. It's a steadfast companion, a stream of life-giving water on a long hike.

Ketoacidosis

Ketoacidosis (Diabetic Ketoacidosis, DKA): A serious condition where the body produces excess blood acids (ketones), often due to insufficient insulin. It's a storm that demands refuge and rapid response.

Metabolic Syndrome

Metabolic Syndrome: A cluster of conditions that occur together, increasing the risk of heart disease, stroke, and diabetes. It's a reminder that the body is an interconnected temple, revealing the importance of holistic maintenance.

Prediabetes

Prediabetes: A state where blood sugar levels are elevated but not high enough to be classified as diabetes. Consider it a measured caution, an invitation to steer the ship with greater care.

As we conclude this glossary, let it be a garden where you may harvest understanding and nourishment. May you find in these terms not only definitions but stepping stones on the path to living in harmony with your body's rhythms. Each word holds the promise of a healthier tomorrow, a foundation upon which to build a resilient spirit.